Arthritis in hands and fingers.

Arthritis in Hands and Fingers Signs, Symptoms, Exercises, Treatment, Pain Prevention, Diet and much more.

by

Lucy Rudford

Published by Zoodoo Publishing 2024

Table of Contents

Chapter 1) Introduction

Humanity has fought with pain and suffering from the very beginning of its existence. The severity of a disease was always evaluated against the devastating pain it caused. Ancient Egyptian manuscripts repeatedly refer to painful diseases descending upon kings, queens and commoners. One particular king, King Ra had severe debilitating episodes of head pain and tried almost all the big names in medicine of the time. Things changed with time as medical science progressed and newer treatments helped in controlling pain thresholds, but total control remained an illusion.

In recent history, Thomas Sydenham, a renowned English physician, produced a detailed account of his sufferings from gout pain for more than three decades. The two world wars saw a huge number of amputees and wounded soldiers experiencing almost every type of traumatic pain. Even today, when medical science has achieved a lot in terms of improving the quality of life, it is very common for ordinary people to experience the physical, emotional, social and economic effects of painful diseases.

Of all the painful conditions, the pain of arthritis in hands and feet is responsible for lowering quality of life and inducing disabilities both temporary and permanent. The NHS has estimated the self reported arthritis to be around 60% for people aged above 60 years. The problem gets worse here, because a good number of people over 50 years of age have some other medical condition, in addition to arthritis. It is important to note that arthritis is not the disease of old age only. A study conducted by the National Institute of Health USA has shown that arthritis and other musculoskeletal disorders are responsible for disability in the majority of people aged 16 to 72 years. This is further established by the fact that only heart diseases have a higher incidence of work disability and arthritis comes in at a close second place. The prevalence of arthritis increases with increase in age, still more than 60% of arthritis sufferers are in their working years of life. This not only dispels this wrong perception that arthritis is a disease of the old; it also establishes the importance of effective treatment and their socio-economic effects.

The major reason for arthritis and its subtypes is a wear and tear in joints. This wear and tear can be: age related as in old people, lifestyle related as in athletes & sportsmen and in response to certain traumatic events like accidents, where a bone or joint is injured.

The most common misconception about *Arthritis* is that it is considered only as a dysfunction for the elderly. But no, this is not the case. Unfortunately, anybody can be affected by arthritis at any stage of his/her life. After a positive diagnosis, the life of a patient takes several new turns. First of all, it is very critical to determine the type of *Arthritis* because several specific steps must be followed for each type. Like in *Polyarticular juvenile Rheumatoid Arthritis*, more than a dozen joints are affected collectively, 28 to be exact in most of the cases. These 28 also include joints of hands and feet. The patient has to seek professional treatment and needs to visit a number of doctors and therapists. Some patients with *Arthritis* are advised to make dietary changes, some are asked to add exercises to their routines and others turn to medication straightaway. These medications are for the sole purpose of easing the pain away and lessening the inflammation in swollen joints. The doctors also have to be careful in order to keep the joints protected so that *Arthritis* should not interfere in the normal growth of the body.

The actual condition and stage of *Arthritis* can only be determined by a qualified physician after proper examination but one should realize that arthritis can hit at any stage. We also need to include interacted drugs while taking medication for *Arthritis* to counter their side effects like nausea, vitamin and mineral deficiencies and abdominal upset.

The good news is that nowadays there are numerous qualified health care providers and amazing physicians that can keep you away from the seemingly inevitable state of moving with the help of a wheelchair; they can keep your body strong. Some of them provide exercise manuals specifically designed for strengthening muscles and keeping the joints flexible. While others make you realize and keep you mentally strong so that you should not quit and commit intentionally to achieve complete recovery. Some other practitioners also suggest that friends and family should accompany the patient, as they might feel bad about their condition and feel hesitant in explaining it to others. Nevertheless, with awareness and proper guidance people feel relaxed and happy to talk about it and to explain it to others.

1) Living with Arthritis:

Living successfully with this disease starts from learning about it as much as you can. Read more and more about it and look for answers to your questions for treatment and preventive options. Consult your physician and prepare an exercise schedule and diet plan. Anyone who has *Arthritis* is certainly not alone but one among millions. In the United States an estimated seventy million people are diagnosed with Arthritis or a related disorder. There are several forms and states of *Arthritis* categorized on severity and course of the ailment. Fortunately, there are several ways to minimize and control the symptoms of Arthritis like exercises, surgeries, joint protection equipments and a number of new drugs are also available for making life easier.

Individuals with *Arthritis* can still receive pleasure and satisfaction through physical activities but they have to take special care of their bodies. Anyone can beat arthritis just by keeping a fully assured attitude and refusing to let it take anything away from your life.

2) Arthritis: What's All this about?

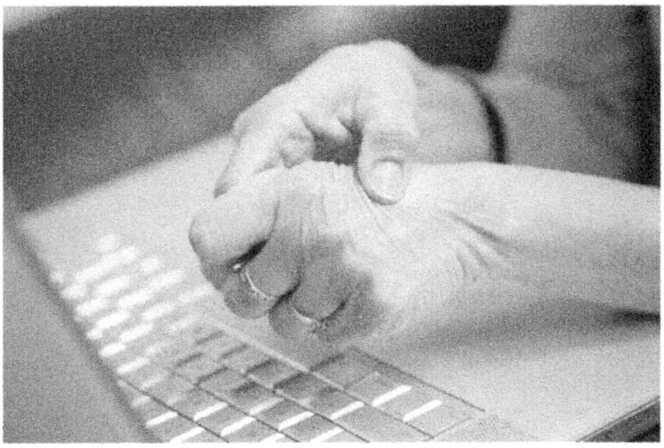

Research and statistics from various sources reveal that around 10% to 20% of people from all ages and genders suffer from one of many types of Arthritis. Many clinicians believe that there are more than 100 types of Arthritis. This number might be an exaggeration but it is true that many types do exist. More than ten types are more common than the rest and nearly 95 percent of patients carry symptoms for these general types. We will view these common types in this book. We will also discuss whether there are conditions that are similar to, and might be confused with, Arthritis. One of these conditions includes an infection called *Lyme disease*. Most physicians opt for antibiotic medications to cure this infection as quickly as possible whenever there are signs of its presence.

This book provides a detailed account of arthritis in hands and feet with a structured approach to ensure that a variety of aspects are explained.

Chapter 2) Pain & Rheumatic Diseases

There are so many different types of arthritis that it's very difficult to explain each and every one. Either as a patient or as a treatment provider, focus usually remains on managing pain and the severity of symptoms, irrespective of the type of arthritis. Pain is something common to all arthritis types including arthritis localized to hands and fingers. In 2012, there were 43 million people in the United States alone suffering from some type of arthritis. This scenario is going to be a far bigger problem for healthcare providers by the end of 2020 when there will be 60 million people suffering from arthritis. These are conservative projections; some healthcare organizations are expecting this number to be doubled by the end of 2021. "*Recent surveys by the Centers for Disease Control and Prevention suggest that 33% (69.9 million) of the U.S. population is affected by arthritis or joint disorders*".

There are two other important factors that are contributing to the rise in prevalence of arthritis. One of these factors is obesity and the other is an increase in the average age in the developed countries. Obese people have more weight on their joints, while old population have a weak immune system and bones. Both of these scenarios are estimated to get worse and by 2020 the osteoarthritis prevalence in the US will increase from 66% to 100%.

What we learn from these projections is very important and will create a significant impact on the shape and structure of our healthcare system. If it is imminent that we are going to see a surge in the prevalence of arthritis to a magnitude of 60 million

Americans, then we must be prepared to tackle it as common household diseases like fever and cold. Unfortunately, this is not the case. Most Americans are unaware of the medical, social, financial and psychological consequences of arthritis. Their knowledge about the disease is limited to Non Steroidal Anti-Inflammatory Drugs and their side effects. Few others know about medical complications and effects on the quality of life. Only those who actually suffer from it realize the huge impact it creates on their lives. This is only a part of the overall problem. The major problem lies with the health professionals. The majority of health professionals simply don't know how to manage chronic pain. There are very few medical schools in the United States that have proper pain courses in their syllabuses. The courses that are available through other professional organizations are taken up by a very select few. This results in inappropriate management of the arthritic pain as doctors are not properly equipped to tackle it. Things just didn't stop there; the last decade has witnessed a lot of bad pain management cases.

In this chapter we will look into the definitions of arthritic pain, what factors affect it, how it can be reduced and finally its effects on your body.

1) Pain

According to the Merriam Webster Medical dictionary, pain is "*a state of physical, emotional, or mental lack of well-being or physical, emotional, or mental uneasiness that ranges from mild discomfort or dull distress to acute often unbearable agony, may be generalized or localized, and is the consequence of being injured or hurt physically or mentally or of some derangement of or lack of equilibrium in the physical or mental functions (as through disease), and that usually produces a reaction of wanting to avoid, escape, or destroy the causative factor and its effects*".

All the parameters of the above definition are applicable to arthritic pain. It affects the patient both physically and mentally, it creates a feeling of uneasiness, it may lead to depression, it deprives him/her of a balanced life and he/she wants to get rid of it at all costs. Pain is one of the first few symptoms to appear in arthritis of the hand and fingers. Initially, this pain may be subtle or dull, but it increases in severity as the disease progresses. Sometimes it is coupled with a burning sensation in the wrist and finger joints. The onset of pain occurs usually either after prolonged use of the joints or prolonged rest. Morning pain and stiffness is a typical example of pain after prolonged rest of the joints. The pain after using the joints may not appear instantly, but can appear after a few hours or maybe the next day. This time usually reduces as the disease progresses and the cartilage wears down.

2) Factors Affecting Pain Severity

There are certain factors that affect the pain severity, like gender, family history, localization and ethnicity.

Males are less tolerant to pain compared to females. This is partially attributed to sex hormones. The male hormone testosterone is associated with an increased pain threshold in animal studies in comparison to the female hormone estrogen. Women also recover more quickly from painful disorders compared to men.

Family history and the upbringing of each individual are reflected in his/her pain perception. Children who are given extraordinary care in response to mild injuries tend to feel pain more severely. Those who are ignored at such minor injuries tend to feel less severity.

Localization of the pain can also affect its severity. Pain in vital and more frequently used organs is felt more than in other, non-vital and less used organs. The example is that pain in the head is more disturbing and severe than pain in the outer ear. Similarly, pain in the hand is more severe than pain in the legs.

Ethnicity and cultural backgrounds play a vital role in developing pain perceptions. Individuals from rural areas tend to have a higher tolerance for pain compared to the urban population. The effect of different ethnic and cultural backgrounds is under investigation for different diseases including arthritis and many more revelations are expected when the results will come from these research studies.

3) How to reduce the pain

This can be achieved via certain exercises, medications and in some cases via surgical treatment. Knuckle Bend and Fist Stretch are very good at easing hand or wrist pain. We'll discuss in detail the different therapeutic approaches in the coming chapters.

Chapter 3) Arthritis & Musculoskeletal Disorders

Arthritis is a specific term used for pain and inflammation in joints of various parts of our body that include the joints of hands, feet, legs, shoulders, neck, back and hips. We have already discussed pain in detail so now we can focus on a few other symptoms. Morning stiffness or aching should not be considered as Arthritis, although it can be one of the manifestations of different arthritis types. Additionally, aching is not always the main symptom of Arthritis. Several other symptoms can indicate the presence of arthritis like tenderness, stiffness, redness, swelling and unnatural warmth in muscles, joints and tissues nearby. The severity of the swelling, stiffness and aching may vary from moderate to serious levels but generally Arthritis is painful. This pain can cause permanent disability in the case of unattended or delayed treatment. Serious types of disabilities are mostly related to Arthritis in the hands and feet. Even minor delays can result in long term limitations in working because hands and fingers are among the most frequently used organs of the body. In order to better understand arthritis and its consequences, we need to learn a few things about joints, their types and their movements.

1) What is a Joint?

Every two bones of our body meet at a particular point that is called a joint. All body movements are possible due to our joints. These joints keep the skeleton together and provide flexibility and range of motion.

2) Types of Joints

Three main types of joints are known that include immovable (fibrous) joints, partially moveable (cartilaginous) joints and the third type is completely moveable (Synovial) joints.

Immovable (fibrous) joints: These types of joints do not show any movement. Our skull contains several immovable joints.

Cartilaginous Joints: Some joints in our body are not completely moveable but do show movement to a limited extend. The Sacroiliac joint in the pelvis is an appropriate example of this joint. The Sacroiliac joint allows spring type movement when we walk and run. A humans' vertebral column is also linked with small cartilaginous joints.

Synovial Joints: Unlike the two other types, these joints are flexible and possess comprehensive movement mechanisms. Synovial joints are present throughout our body in all shapes and sizes. Hands, fingers, shoulders, elbows, wrists, knees, ankles and hips are all included in freely moveable joints. We will concentrate more on the joints of hands and fingers in this book.

3) Joints of hands and fingers

The joints of hands and fingers are some of the most significant synovial joints of our body that are used more than any other joint of the body. They also provide the maximum range of movement when compared to other joints.

The structure of synovial joints consists of five parts:

-*Synovium*-it produces a fluid-type secretion that provides lubrication, enabling joints to move freely.

-*Joint Capsule*-it is the outer most part of a joint that keeps it safe like a bag and maintains its shape.

-*Cartilage*-it is more of a shock absorber that hides the ends of two connecting bones.

-*Ligaments*-it is a fold of membranes that holds two bones together.

-*Tendons*-tendons are strong cords that keep the joint in place by attaching muscles to the bones on either side.

Now that we have understood the basics about joints, particularly about the joints of the hands and fingers, we can easily move along with further, in-depth information about Arthritis in hands and fingers.

4) Pathophysiology-Arthritic Hands and Arthritic Fingers

The basic pathophysiology of all types of Arthritis including arthritic hands and fingers revolves around joint wear and tear, although the underlying conditions may be different for some of them. Cartilage degeneration is involved in Osteoarthritis (OA). The cartilage endures a remodeling process triggered by joint movement. However, in OA this situation is changed by a number of reasons including cellular, mechanical and biochemical processes that lead to the reduction of the efficacy, strength and diminution of cartilage. As the disease worsens, new bones at joint margins might develop with an increase in thickness of the sub-chondral plate. In progression, this can lead to a severe deterioration of the cartilage. The mechanism of RA is different in a way that rheumatoid arthritis is an autoimmune disease.

Ulcers, genetic problems, environmental disturbances and hormonal disorders are the basic factors that may trigger RA. It can either be due to an initial response of the immune system's inflammatory cytokines or the production of autoantibodies. These two create a sequence of inflammation due to the formation of pannus (proliferation of synovial tissue). This pannus makes a forceful entry to the joint, resulting in damage of the cartilage and subsequently the bones. RA is also related to hormonal disturbances so it is more common in females than males, especially during pregnancy, when the chances of its onset are relatively high.

5) Perception & Assessment

Pain associated with arthritis in hands and fingers is a subjective experience that cannot be observed or measured directly. The severity of pain is not a standard scale to underline the progression of disease. In fact, in some experiences the patient is unaware to the worsening of their symptoms due to lack of pain.

6) Rating Scales

Professional and self-administered measurements in arthritic hands or arthritic fingers consist of several factors and norms. These factors include physical activity, pain, mobility, dexterity and household activities; walking and bending, hands and fingers functioning, social activities, physical activities like weight lifting, degree of anxiety and level of depression.

7) Arthritic Hands & Fingers Associated Pain in Old Age

The chances of Arthritis in hands and fingers and associated pain increase with age. Most patients neglect the pain, as it can be normal for the old, especially those above 65 years. With age, the senses of smell, taste and sensation are weakened but the pain, aching and daily routine activities due to arthritic hands and fingers can cause serious difficulties.

8) Hands & Fingers Arthritis in Youngsters

Sadly, Arthritis in hands and fingers is not limited to the elderly. Youngsters can develop symptoms of arthritis as well. Beulah was a beautiful 23-year-old, young, working lady. She was successful and happily married to Clifford. They were planning to start a family and have kids. They were truly in love and were living the American dream with a clear focus on their prosperous future. Unfortunately, one day Beulah started to feel swelling and stiffness in her hands and fingers. In only a few days' time the same feeling of aching and pain spread to her hips, ankles, knees, elbows, shoulders and feet. There was so much swelling in her fingers that she was unable to perform even easy routine tasks.

The onset of arthritis in hands and fingers is usually quick, with severe symptoms. These symptoms rapidly increase in severity, resulting in partial disability.

9) How common it is?

The Arthritis Foundation has researched Arthritic hands and fingers as a leading cause of disability in United Stated of America. There are about 3.75 million females and 1.5 million males who have Arthritis in the hands or fingers. *[Arthritis Rheum 2010 Jun;62(6):1576-82. [Data Source: Patient Cohort,*

Minnesota]. Work limitations resulting from Arthritic hands and Arthritic fingers are at about 31% among all types of Arthritic disorders.

Chapter 4) Types of Arthritis and Rheumatic Diseases

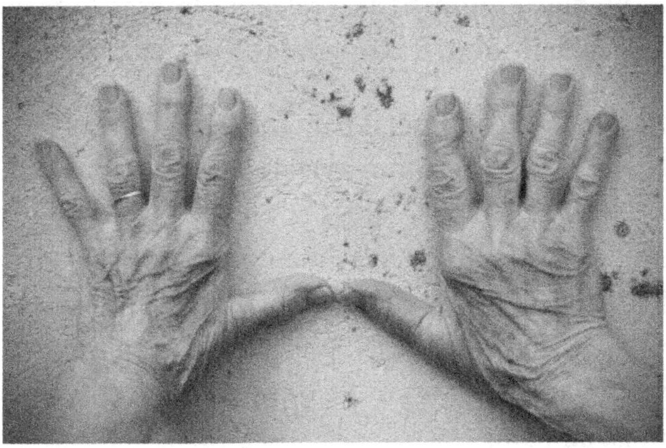

Arthritis is the most common degenerative bone disease in old age and may affect both genders equally in their early 40's. It is interesting to know that there are different types of arthritis; in fact, more than 100 types of arthritis are known. All have different symptoms and different treatments. Arthritis may affect one or more joints of different parts of the body on one or both sides. For example, it may affect hands, fingers, the thumb, spine, knee, foot, and backbone. It can cause pain, swelling and stiffness in joints; it may be symmetrical and be present in both hands. It is important for you to learn the major differences among different types of arthritis. There is a need to diagnose the correct type of arthritis so that the damage caused by arthritis to the joints can be controlled as soon as possible. The most **common types** of arthritis are Osteoarthritis, Rheumatoid arthritis and Gouty arthritis.

1) Myofascial Pain:

Myofascial pain syndrome is a chronic pain disorder in which muscles and tissues of the face develop trigger points. These trigger points can be painful when poked but they cause pain in another, unrelated part of the body. This pain is called referred pain. These trigger points are formed as a result of trauma to that tissue. They cause pain and strain throughout the muscle.

a) ***Sign and symptoms*** of Myofascial pain include: a tender knot in the muscle, deep aching pain in muscles, the pain that persists and get worse slowly due to stress or any physical activity, tinnitus and ear pain, headaches, memory problems, migraine and difficulty sleeping due to pain. Unexplained nausea, numbness in extremities, clicking joints, blurred vision and limited range of motion of the joints of the jaw are other specific symptoms of myofascial pain.

b) Diagnosis of myofascial pain syndrome is done through physical examinations. Doctors may apply gentle pressure with their fingers to the painful area to find the trigger points. A tissue biopsy and Magnetic resonance elastography can be used to show the abnormalities in trigger points but they are not confirmatory tests for myofascial pain syndrome.

c) Treatment options for Myofascial pain syndrome include physical therapy, medications and trigger point injections. In the case of medication, pain relievers, sedatives and anti-depressants are used. In physical therapy, massage, stretching exercises and heat application via a hot pack can be done to reduce pain and muscle tension. With Acupuncture, needle procedures are also used to inject numbing agent or steroid into the trigger points. Dry needling is also used to relieve pain in myofascial pain syndrome.

More than one option can be used according to the severity of the disease.

2) Fibromyalgia:

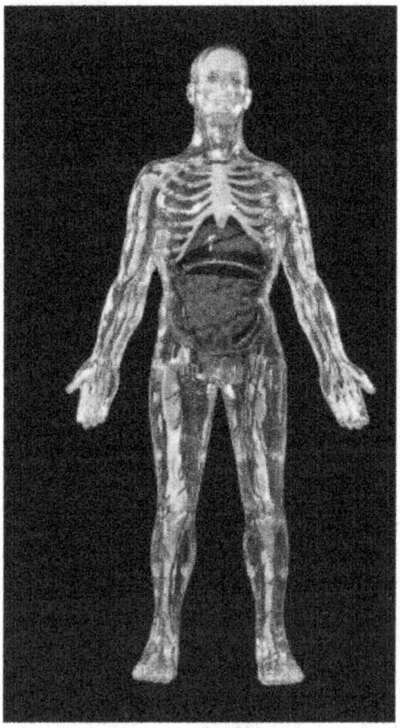

This is characterized by the musculoskeletal pain that is accompanied by mood issues, sleep and memory issues and fatigue. Fibromyalgia exaggerates the pain sensation by affecting the processing of pain signals in the brain. The pain associated with fibromyalgia is a constant dull ache; additional pain when pressure is applied to the tender points of the body is also a characteristic of Fibromyalgia.

Locations of tender points include: the front side of the neck, top of the shoulders, between the shoulder blades, back of the head, the outer elbow, upper chest, sides of hips, upper hips and the inner knee.

a) ***Symptoms*** of Fibromyalgia are: fatigue, allergies and sensitivities, confusion and disorientation, and panic attacks. Anxiety, headaches, endometriosis, depression and irritable bowel syndrome are other symptoms. People with fibromyalgia have a long period of sleep but they often awake tired. Sleep is disturbed by pain resulting in sleep apnea, restless legs syndrome, and a further worsening of symptoms.

b) Causes of fibromyalgia could be genetic mutation as it runs in the family, but also some infection or physical trauma can also trigger the fibromyalgia.

c) Diagnosis of fibromyalgia is difficult as symptoms of fibromyalgia come and go, but according to the current guidelines, the criteria for the diagnosis of fibromyalgia include:

- Widespread pain lasting for at least three months
- No other underlying condition causing pain

There is no lab test to confirm the diagnosis of fibromyalgia.

d) Treatment of fibromyalgia includes self-care and medications. Medications that are used in treating fibromyalgia are anti-seizure, analgesics, and antidepressants. NSAIDs are not effective in treating fibromyalgia because they target inflammation, and it is not an inflammatory disease.

Studies have shown that trigger point injections are also not effective in relieving the tender points in fibromyalgia so they are not used either. Counseling can be helpful to guide you about different strategies to deal with stress and to strengthen your belief in your abilities.

It is interesting that fibromyalgia and myofascial pain syndrome often go together and have so many common symptoms, but they are two different problems as their treatment plan is different, and treating myofascial pain syndrome can help in calming fibromyalgia.

3) Osteoarthritis:

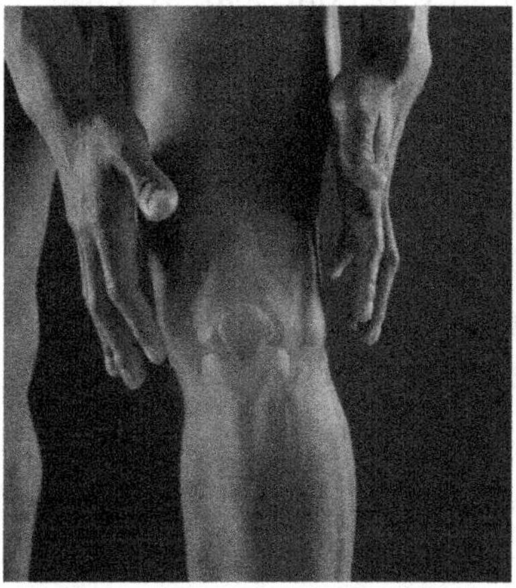

It is the most common type of arthritis, often called wear and tear arthritis. Osteoarthritis can damage any joint of your body and it has no cure, and it deteriorates gradually with time. It is a less aggressive form of arthritis and it progresses slowly. It is diagnosed more in men below 45 and in women above 45 years of age.

a) ***Symptoms*** of osteoarthritis are loss of flexibility, pain, joint tenderness, grating sensation, bone spur, joint stiffness etc.

***b) Causes*:** Cartilage is a firm tissue that allows frictionless joint movement but in OA, the surface of cartilage becomes rough with time and it eventually wears down, resulting in the rubbing of a bone with another bone.

***c) Diagnosis*:** After physical examination and assessing the patient history, an X-ray test can be used to know the degree of joint damage. A joint aspiration test may also help in diagnosis.

d) Treatment options for OA include medications (acetaminophen, narcotics and NSAIDs), physical therapy, and occupational therapy, surgical and other procedures as well as special bracing of the hands and fingers to support them.

***e) Clinical presentation*:** Osteoarthritis mostly affects distal interphalangeal (DIP) joints of hands but may also involve proximal interphalangeal (PIP) joints and the joints at the base of the thumb. Heber den nodes are more common in females than males and represent the palpable osteophytes in DIP joints of hands.

4) Rheumatoid Arthritis:

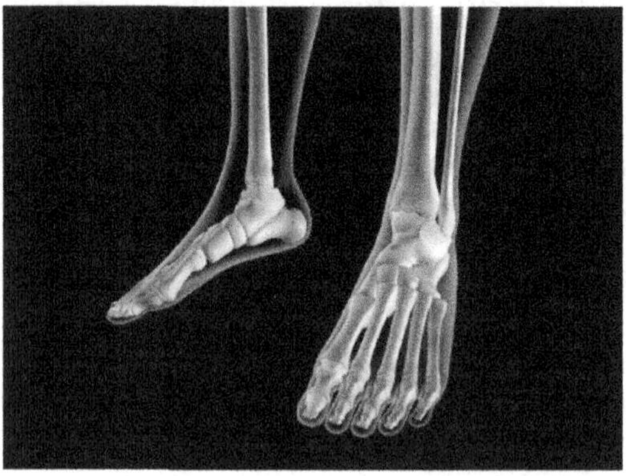

It is one of the most common types of arthritis and is a chronic inflammatory disorder that affects the lining of small joints of the hands and feet, resulting in painful swelling with bone erosion and eventual joint deformity. It is an autoimmune disorder and occurs when the body's immune system starts attacking the body's own tissues. It usually begins after the age of 40 but can occur at any age.

***a) Symptoms*:** Symptoms of rheumatoid arthritis may vary in severity and may come and go; a period with active symptoms of the disease is called flare and a relaxed period is called remission. Morning stiffness, tenderness, painful, inflamed joints with fever, fatigue and weight loss are common symptoms of rheumatoid arthritis.

Rheumatic nodules are the firm lumps located under the skin and grow close to the affected joints. These nodules may have no pain in some cases but could be painful for many people. They may interfere with daily activities and may limit the mobility of effected joints. Rheumatic nodules usually occur in patients with severe Rheumatoid arthritis having a positive rheumatoid factor test. Disease-modifying anti-rheumatic drugs (DMARDs) can be used to reduce the size of the nodules.

***b) Diagnosis*:** It is difficult to diagnose using a single test in the early stages. During physical examination, swelling, redness and warmth are observed. X-rays may help to know the progression of RA over time. Increased ESR rate indicates the inflammatory process. Other blood tests for diagnosis are rheumatoid factor (RF) and anti-cyclic citrullinated peptide (anti-CCP).

***c) Treatment*:** There is no cure for RA, but treatment is given to reduce the inflammation and pain. Medication is usually combined with physical and occupational therapy for this purpose. Medication involves the usage of NSAIDs, TNF-alpha inhibitors, steroids, DMARDs, immunosuppressant and some others. Sometimes surgery can also be carried out if medications fail to prevent or slow the rate of joint damage.

***d) Clinical presentation*:** In RA of the fingers, the metacarpal joints may begin to point sideways towards the little finger, known as *ulnar drift*. This drift causes pain and weakness in joints and deformity becomes evident, making daily activities difficult. The *boutonniere deformity* of fingers shows hyperextension of the distal interphalangeal (DIP) joint of the finger along with non-reducible flexion at the PIP joint of the finger. This joint deformity occurs as a result of a rupturing of the PIP joint or stretching of synovitis. Complications of boutonniere deformity are pincher grasp and loss of thumb mobility. *Swan-neck deformity* of the fingers describes flexion of the DIP joint and hyperextension at the PIP joint.

In meta-carpophalangeal joints, two deformities that alter the stability of fingers and alignment of palmal skeletal arches are *volar sub-luxation* and *ulnar deviation.*

5) Psoriatic Arthritis:

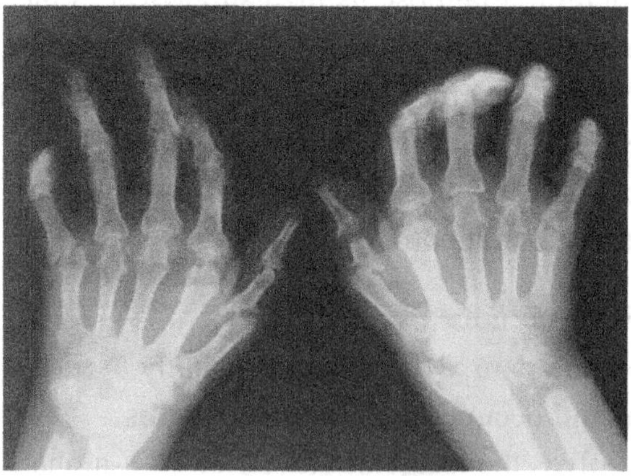

It is the form of arthritis that affects people who have psoriasis, which is a skin problem producing red patches of the skin with silvery scales. They can affect any part of your body, including the spine, fingertips and hands with mild to severe intensity. There is no cure for psoriatic arthritis but without treatment it may become disabling. It usually strikes around age 30-50.

a) ***Symptoms***: Painful joints that are swollen and cause pain when touched are the most common symptoms. Sausage-like swelling of fingers and toes is very common. It may cause pain at points where ligaments and tendons are attached with the bones. Lower back pain with inflammation of joints between vertebras of the spine is also present in Psoriatic arthritis.

b) Causes: It occurs when the immune system of the body starts attacking healthy cells of the body, causing inflammation of joints as well as increased production of skin cells. Physical trauma may also trigger the psoriatic arthritis and certain genetic markers are also associated with the psoriatic arthritis.

c) Diagnosis: No single test can assure the diagnosis of psoriatic arthritis, but different tests are used to rule out other causes of pain including RA, and gout. Tests include X-rays and MRI used to check the problems in joints and in tendons in your feet and lower back. Joint fluid tests and RF tests may also help in diagnosis.

d) Treatment: There is no cure for psoriatic arthritis so it is treated only to control the inflammation of the affected joints. The treatment plan involves medications; including Nonsteroidal anti-inflammatory drugs (NSAIDs), disease modifying anti-rheumatic drugs (DMARDs), TNF-alpha inhibitors, and immunosuppressant medicines.

6) Septic Arthritis:

It is an intense, painful infection of joints caused by germs that travel from another part of the body through the blood stream. Penetrating injury into the joint may also cause septic arthritis. The most commonly affected joints are the knee joint and hips and old people and infants are more likely to develop septic arthritis. It is very important to treat septic arthritis as soon as possible because it quickly and severely damages the bone and cartilage within joints.

a) Symptoms: The most common symptoms of septic arthritis are fever with painful swollen joints and experiencing extreme difficulty in using the affected joints.

b) Cause: It may develop due to infection in any other part of the body such as urinary tract infection or upper respiratory tract infection and spreads through the bloodstream to the joint. Open wounds, surgery in or near the joint and drug injection are other sources of infection in septic arthritis.

The lining of joints has the ability to protect itself from infection but reaction of the body towards infection may contribute to the damage of the joint.

c) Diagnosis: Imaging tests, blood tests to check the presence of bacteria in the blood and joint fluid analysis to discover which bacteria is causing infection are the tools used for the diagnosis of septic arthritis.

d) Treatment: The treatment plan for Septic arthritis includes antibiotic drugs and joint drainage. Removing the infected fluid from the joint is crucial so drainage methods are used.

7) What types of arthritis affect the hands?

There are different types of arthritis and how they present themselves in hands is very different. The most common type affecting hands and fingers is osteoarthritis. Rheumatoid arthritis is another type of arthritis that affects the hands. Gouty arthritis can also affect hands but it is more common in feet. Treatment of all these types is different, with different kinds of medications that help in making the condition comfortable. In arthritis of the hands, the most frequently affected joints are small end joints of the fingers.

Chapter 5) Arthritis: Signs, Symptoms & Diagnosis

1) Early Onset signs

Arthritis is a painful condition with many types and affects many parts of the body including hands, fingers, thumb, knee, hipbone etc. All the types of Arthritis have some specific symptoms that are related to each specific type of arthritis. But few of the symptoms of Arthritis are common in all types of Arthritis affecting any type of joint including hands and fingers. Those are pain, joint stiffness (with limited movement of the joints), joint tenderness, and redness (with warmth and swelling at the arthritic joints of hands and fingers).

a) Joint Pain: It is the most common sign of arthritis and it is seldom absent from any inflamed joint. Initially, this pain in joints may become worse after certain activities but it relieves after rest. In some types of arthritis, joint pain is described as a strong burning sensation rather than a sharp pain.

b) Limited Mobility: This is limited mobility of one or more joints that shows the presence of arthritis. It might result in difficulty in dealing with daily tasks. You need to observe whether this is dominant with stretching of the joint or bending of the joint.

c) Joint Stiffness: It is usually felt early in the morning, but it is decreased slowly with time as your body gets involved in different tasks and the movements of joints are increased throughout the day.

d) Joint Tenderness: It should be considered as sign of arthritis if your joints are painful to touch. Tenderness may come and go or it may be consistent, depending on the type and severity of arthritis.

e) Redness and Warmth: It is another sign of arthritis that is caused by inflammation at the site of the arthritic joint. This could be especially present in Rheumatoid arthritis, but it is also present in many other types of arthritis.

Other signs and symptoms of Arthritis include fatigue, weight loss, fever, rashes and many others. Some signs are specific to the type of Arthritis.

2) More Specified Symptoms

There are many other specified symptoms that include aching muscles, tendinitis, joint destruction and then finally joint disability. If arthritis damaged the joint once, then treating inflammation does not return the joint to its original state. This inflammation of soft tissues can result in severe deformity of the joints that will eventually limit the ability of patients to use their hands. Patients of arthritis will experience other systemic symptoms like malaise, loss of appetite and fatigue. These symptoms of Arthritis will manifest differently in different patients.

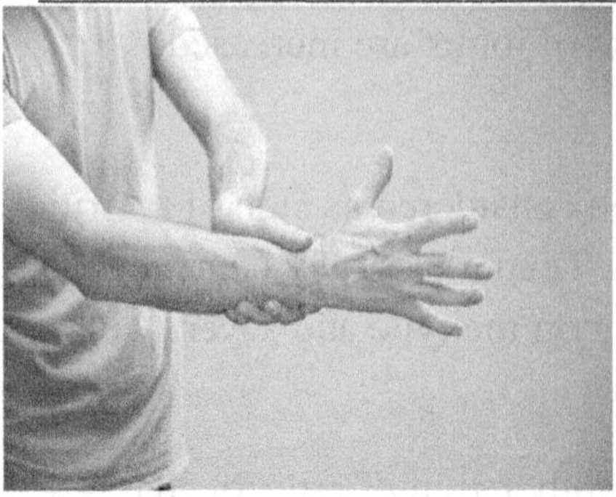

In *rheumatoid arthritis*, with all the symptoms above mentioned, bumps of tissues called rheumatoid nodules are also present under the skin of your fingers. Other symptoms that should not be ignored by Rheumatoid arthritic patients are: inability to move or raise your hand, tingling or numbness of hands, chest pain or shortness of breath, red and inflamed eyes, and spots on and around your fingertips. Numbness and tingling in the joints of hands and fingers are due to swelling in the arm that compresses the nerves going into the hands and it is worse at night. Morning stiffness of joints of hands and fingers is common with rheumatoid arthritis. The difference between morning stiffness caused by OA and RA is the duration, as it is for longer in rheumatoid arthritic patients. Night sweats, sudden weight loss, loss of energy and bone fracture are other symptoms associated with Rheumatoid arthritis. One other interesting feature of rheumatoid arthritis is that pain in joints is symmetrical, that is, both sides of the body parts are affected at a time (both hands, both knees etc.).

In *Osteoarthritis*, the most common sign is joint pain; joints feel tender even when light pressure is applied. Morning stiffness is very common in osteoarthritic patients but it can also occur after a period of inactivity. Joints affected by arthritis cannot be moved easily with their full range of movement and you may feel a grating sensation when those joints are used. Extra bits of bones called bone spurs may form around the effected joint of hands and fingers, which feel like a hard hump.

In *gouty arthritis*, the most common sign is the swelling of joints at nighttime, redness, tenderness and sharp pain in your big toe. It could also attack the knee, ankle, or foot. The attack of gouty arthritis may last for a few days or many weeks. This gout attack is due to the deposition of uric acid in the joints so consult your doctor as soon as possible as it may harm your joints.

3) Hands & Fingers Arthritis in Males/Females

Hands and fingers Arthritis can occur at any age in both genders. Osteoarthritis is the common type of arthritis and is common among females. Rheumatoid arthritis is an autoimmune disease that primarily affects females three times more than males. The incidence of arthritis of different types may vary according to the joints involved. For example, osteoarthritis of the hip is more common in males than females, but degenerative changes of the knee and hand joints are common among females. Gouty arthritis is common among males and infectious arthritis incidence can occur in any gender. Autoimmune diseases are common more in females, like Lupus, for example.

If we discuss the prevalence of arthritis in hands according to gender then RA is approximately 10%, Radiographic OA in wrist and finger joints is 65% and in knee joints it is 14%. Involvement of the first metacarpophalangeal joint of the hand in arthritis is more common in males than females and the enlargement of proximal and distal interphalangeal finger joints are common among females rather than males. This difference is due to the degree of heavy work done in males and females. The prevalence of chondrocalcinosis of hands is about 21% in females but does not exist in males. To conclude the discussion, we can say that the prevalence of arthritis is more common in females. Incidences of arthritis in females are increasing with time; it is 54 per 100,000, and for men it is stable at 29 per 100,000 in the previous ten years.

The reasons why incidences of arthritis of hands and fingers are common in females than males include: Genetic factors affecting specific triggers of arthritis, activity level, obesity, sex based differences in anatomy and neuromuscular development affecting joints, social factors, injury and sex hormone influence. The increased incidence of arthritis in females can also be related to the sex-based differences in anatomy as well as collagen metabolism. Then the ability of women and men to compensate for any functional losses due to difference in bone mineral density, in muscle strength, skin thickness and difference in bone mineral density are other reasons of making Arthritis more common in females.

Another theory about the development of hands and fingers arthritis being common in women is associated with the changes in sex hormone levels including progesterone and estrogen. It is because these hormones have an important role in the inflammatory response and also in the overall regulation of the immune system of the body. These hormones may affect adrenal and thyroid systems, which in turn affect immunity in every cell. They have a direct impact on the cartilage that cushions the area between the bones of the joints, thus protecting bones from rubbing and causing pain against each other. Changes in these hormone levels may also affect protein levels of the body, thus causing an increase in the inflammation process.

Genetic links to arthritis may also be the reason for arthritis as it can run in family history. You may develop arthritis of the same joints at same age as your parents. The female body was designed to have children, that means tendons in her body move and bend more easily than male joints. After menopause, the estrogen levels in the body are reducedand that will contribute to the development of Arthritis of hands and fingers. Stress is also one of the very important factors as it will result in weight gain, depression, eating disorders, and obesity thus affecting the immune function of the body. So stress reduction is very important for health. Regular exercise is the best tool for weight reduction and to control obesity, thus helping in reducing the chances of development of arthritis of hands and fingers.

4) Diagnosis

The doctor carries out the diagnosis of arthritis after physical examination of hands and by taking X-rays. Bone scans may be helpful in the diagnosis of arthritis when it is in an early stage. Arthroscopy is another way to directly inspect the joint condition. It is done by inserting a small camera into the joint to have a clear picture of the joint, however it is an invasive procedure so it should not be used in routine check-ups for diagnosis purposes. Patient history, X-ray results and physical examination findings are used to diagnose arthritis and blood tests are helpful in the case of RA.

It is very important to find out whether you have arthritis and of what type it is, as treatment varies for each type of arthritis. However, this is not an easy task as many types of arthritis have similar or overlapping symptoms in the early stages. With proper diagnosis, you will understand the cause of pain and then further appropriate steps can be taken to relieve the pain. Only a doctor can tell what type of arthritis you have. Doctors may move the joint that hurts to see its range of motion and check for tender points, swelling, skin rashes or other problems associated with arthritis.

Laboratory tests may include a joint fluid test, blood test, urine test, X-rays or scans and muscles tests depending on what type of arthritis the doctor suspects. An overall result from laboratory tests, medical history and physical examination helps your doctor match your symptoms for a specific type of arthritis. It may take time to confirm the type of arthritis as many types of arthritis have slow progression.

5) Significance of Timely Diagnosis

Early diagnosis of arthritis with confirmation of the type of arthritis and planning of treatment based on such an early diagnosis is very important and beneficial for the patient. It will help in preventing joint damage and in slowing the progression of the disease, which is very common during the first few years of Arthritis of hands and fingers.

6) Classification of Propositions

Pain management is most important in arthritic patients as it affects their quality of life and makes daily activities more difficult. Different methods are used for reducing pain. The most common approaches include heat therapy, cold therapy and electrical stimulation. Different products are available for this purpose, but the following are the basic methods:

a) Heat and Cold: Heat is used to reduce muscle spasms as well as pain to help in the stretching of soft tissues and to stimulate blood flow. It is the most commonly used method to reduce pain in joints of fingers and hands affected by arthritis. To apply heat, you can use a warm, damp towel or moist heating pads. A hot tub is also a good option for relaxing muscle stiffness but avoid a hot tub if you are pregnant or a B.P patient. Cold therapy is also used by patients with Arthritis of hands and fingers. It is very useful in the initial treatment of inflammation caused by soft tissue injury and muscle spasms as well as other musculoskeletal disorders including arthritis of the hands and fingers. Hot/cold packs are available for this purpose. You can heat the packs in the microwave or in hot water, but don't go too hot to avoid skin burning. And you can cool them in the fridge or freezer. An ice pack or cool compress can also be used on the affected joint to help in reducing the pain and inflammation. Avoid long exposure and apply a cold compress only for 15 minutes at a time with a break of 30 minutes between the sessions.

b) Electrical stimulation*:* Electricity can be used to help in reducing pain and swelling in arthritic joints in different ways. In Electro-acupuncture, needles are used at acupuncture points that are attached to electrodes to pass an electric charge through acupuncture needles. In physical therapy, transcutaneous electro-stimulation is carried out, which involves electrodes around the affected joints to pass electromagnetic pulses through the skin. Both of these approaches help in providing short-term pain relief and also reduce the joint stiffness in arthritis of hands and fingers.

Chapter 6) Medical Treatments

1) Surgery

Surgery is the last possible option in treatment of arthritis and is usually reserved for severe arthritis that does not respond to other arthritis treatments and also limits your activities significantly. However, surgery is recommended before arthritis causes muscle loss and joint deformities. Patients after surgery should be kept in the best possible physical conditions.

There are many surgical options including: Synovectomy, Arthroscopy, Joint Irrigation, Joint fusion, Realignment and joint replacement and cartilage grafting. *Synovectomy* is the removal of destructive tissues. Sometimes these tissues are tightened around the joint to provide relief as this disease causes loosening of the tissues around the joint.

If the joint is completely destroyed then joint replacement or joint fusion are effective options. In *joint replacement therapy,* the joint is replaced with an artificial joint (silicone implant or metal). It is very effective in older and less active individuals and it dramatically decreases the pain, lasting for at least 3 years. *Joint Fusion* or making the joint solid is an effective treatment option of thumb metacarpal arthritis. It is recommended for those joints that are badly damaged but for which joint replacement surgery is not appropriate. Fusion is recommended usually for joints of the wrist and for small joints of fingers. Long-standing arthritis may cause misalignment of the bones and joints so *Realignment surgery* may be used to realign the bones and other affected joints. *Cartilage grafting* can be carried out in damaged regions of cartilage. It is done only when cartilage damage is confined to small areas of cartilage, surrounded by normal cartilage. *Arthroscopy* involves tissue repair inside the joint through small openings in the skin and is useful for repairing torn cartilage.

The specific procedure that is selected for treatment depends on the type of that particular joint involved, the condition of the surrounding joints, the degree of damage and any particular needs of an individual patient. There are many ways to treat deformities of hands in arthritis patients. Problems that occur after any type of surgery are: infection, breakage or loosening of the artificial joint.

2) Surgery-Why and Why Not?

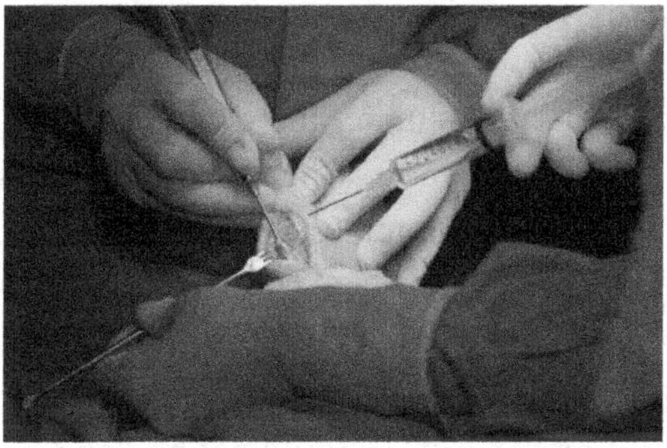

The need for surgery is based on the severity of symptoms, responses to other therapies and the priorities of the individuals.

If more than one joint is affected, it is risky to perform surgery because multilevel fusion is not advisable. So use medications for this purpose.

Advantages of Surgery:

The benefits of surgical procedures include:

- May improve hand functions
- May improve hand appearance
- Possible reduction in pain
- Ability to perform daily activities easily

Disadvantages of Surgery:

The disadvantages of surgery include:

- Replacement joints, for example, new knuckle joints are not as durable as natural joints
- Some operations restrict joint movement
- Other complications of surgery, including infections, may further deteriorate the existing problem.

3) Surgery for rheumatoid nodules

Rheumatoid nodules are the firm lumps under the skin of patients with advanced RA. These nodules appear near the pressure points or the affected joints including hands, knuckles, fingers and elbows. Sometimes nodules disappear and heal spontaneously without any treatment but sometimes surgical removal is required. They do not disfigure the patient at all so it is the individual's choice to surgically remove it or not, but it should not be done until the nodules become infected or start to limit mobility or there is a significant level of discomfort.

a) Symptoms of Nodules: The size and placing of nodules have effects on the symptoms as some patients have no pain whatsoever from the presence of nodules. However, when nodules are located near nerves it will result in constant pain and limit the range of motion if nodules are on the joints.

b) Diagnosis of Nodules: Diagnosis is made clinically, some laboratory tests are also useful, as rheumatoid nodules need to be differentiated from fibromas, gouty tophi, xanthomas, synovial cysts, nodular scleroderma and metastatic tumors.

c) Treatment: Injections of certain drugs including Hydroxy-chloriquine and corticosteroids are effective means of treating these nodules by decreasing their size and eliminating them. DMARDs tend to reduce the size of nodules and also the likelihood of their formation again. The exception is Methotrexate as it increases the number of nodules. Surgical removal is a reasonably successful option for nodules and they can be easily excised.

4) Negative aspects of surgical removal of Nodules include:

Surgical removal is not a perfect option for nodules as it is simple but short-term treatment. There is a good chance of reoccurrence of nodules over time, especially the nodules that form over pressure points will re-grow within a few months. Another problem is the use of the Anti-rheumatic drug Methotrexate, as it causes nodules to grow quicker and larger. So you have to eliminate this medication from the therapy. To get funding for treatment of rheumatic nodules is another problem because nodules are not always the source of discomfort or pain and it might be considered a purely cosmetic problem.

5) Common Types of hand surgery

The most common types of hand surgeries are:

- Ganglion removal
- Tendon repair
- Thumb joint surgery

- Trigger finger release
- Carpel tunnel release
- Knuckle (MCP joint) replacement
- Dupuytren's contracture fasciectomy

6) Complementary Therapies

Complementary therapies are helpful for many people with Arthritis of the hands and fingers. They do not cure the disease but only reduce the symptoms. Complementary medicine uses the therapies that can work alongside conventional medicine to have better results.

There are many types of Complementary therapies and all of them can be divided into three categories as:

- Mind and emotion therapies
- Medicine and diet related therapies
- Pressure, touch and movement therapies

Some of the most popular therapies used for arthritis of hands and fingers are: Yoga, Music therapy, Magnet therapy, T'ai chi, Meditation, Hydrotherapy, Homeopathy, Aromatherapy, Massage, Chiropractic, Alexander technique, Osteopathy and Acupuncture, Glucosamine and Chondroitin Supplementation.

a) Acupuncture*:* It involves the insertion of extremely thin needles through the skin at specific points of the hands and fingers. It is the most commonly used method of Traditional Chinese medicine to treat pain. The goal of Acupuncture is to restore the energy known as "qi or chi" that flows in the body. If this energy goes out of balance then it leads to illness and pain. Acupuncture practitioners believe that when needles are inserted at the specific points, this energy flow gets re-balanced.

Western practitioners believe that these special points are the places to stimulate the nerves, connective tissues and muscles. This stimulation leads to the increased blood flow, and enhanced natural painkilling activity. Acupuncture involves stimulating the special points on the hand and fingers through different techniques including the insertion of needles, heat and pressure. It is effective in reducing pain in arthritic joints of hands and fingers. Acupuncture shows an improvement in pain associated with arthritis patients suffering from OA and RA.

The risks associated with this technique are very low if an experienced acupuncture practitioner does it properly. However, possible side effects are soreness at the site of needle insertion on the hands and fingers, and infection that could occur if hygienic measures are not taken during the procedure.

b) Vitamin D: Vitamin D is an important nutrient for strong bones and helps in regulating the immune system of the body and reduces the disease. Vitamin D is required for healthy muscles and strong bones along with Calcium and plays an important role in slowing the progression of Arthritis in hands and fingers. It is essential in calcium metabolism and bone functioning, cartilage repair and stimulation of collagen production. Subjects with low serum levels of 25-hydroxyvitamin D have a three-fold higher risk of radiographic disease prevention. Exposure to sunlight activates Vitamin D synthesis in the body by your skin and is taken in through diet and also through supplementation. The exact therapeutic dose of Vitamin D for arthritis of hands and fingers is not known but the current recommended dose for prevention of Arthritis of hands and fingers is 400-800 I.U. per day.

c) Antioxidants: Free radicals are one of the major reasons in inducing Arthritis of hands and fingers but vitamins, particularly antioxidants, play an important role in preventing Arthritis. Vitamin C is an antioxidant. Antioxidants delay cartilage degeneration and thus prevent the disease from progressing rapidly. Subjects with low serum levels of Vitamin C have a higher risk of developing arthritis of the hands and fingers. This is because Vitamin C is required for the stabilization of mature collagen. Vitamin C exerts its effects on the Vitamin C-dependent enzyme lysyl-hydroxylase for the production of collagen. Collagen is an important component of bones, ligaments and tendons so it will result in the easing of pain and other symptoms. The Recommended Dietary Allowance (RDA) of Vitamin C is 125mg per day.

d) Chondroitin Sulfate: Chondroitin sulfate is a naturally occurring molecule and it is the main component of joint cartilage protein and gives cartilage its elastic properties. It is widely used in alternative therapy for Arthritis of the hands and fingers. It stimulates the production of collagen and proteoglycan and partially inhibits the enzymatic degradation. It relieves morning stiffness, improves hand functioning and eases the pain associated with arthritis. It has anti-inflammatory properties, and helps in reducing painful swelling in joints. It slows down the degradation of cartilage and helps in restoring cartilage growth to cushion the joints better.

Studies have shown that Chondroitin sulfate is safe to use in arthritis patients and have no side effects that are produced by NSAIDs. NSAIDs provide similar pain relieving effects but they have many side effects with long-term toxicities. The effects of treatment with NSAIDs disappear immediately after stopping the treatment but the effects of Chondroitin last for 3 months after therapy discontinuation. Doses of Chondroitin sulfate vary for individual patients but usually 1200mg per day is used for hand arthritis.

e) Glucosamine: It is a salt of D-glucosamine, an amino sugar that contains sulfuric acid. Glucosamine is a dietary supplement and is a safe, natural and non-toxic compound. It is widely used in Arthritis of hands and fingers as it not only stops the pain but also improves the structure of the joint by rebuilding cartilage and reverses the progression of arthritis. Glucosamine is a Chondroprotective agent and relieves the symptoms of Arthritis without any serious side effects. Chondroitin and Glucosamine are naturally produced within the body, but in the case of arthritis, it is not produced in sufficient amounts. That is why it is used as a supplement to replenish our system. Glucosamine is made from shells of shrimp so it should be used with caution in patients that are allergic to shellfish. It may also increase the blood sugar level as it blocks the effects of Insulin so it should be avoided in diabetic patients, nursing and pregnant women.

Glucosamine and Chondroitin sulfate are usually used in combination. They are present in different ratios in different marketed products. Usually 1500mg of Glucosamine and 1200mg of Chondroitin sulfate per day is used to treat Arthritis of hands and fingers.

7) Intra-articular medications

a) Steroid Injections: Steroids are used in the treatment of arthritis, and their effects are short-lived. Glucocorticoid acts at cellular level and inhibits the inflammatory mediators and controls the synthesis of various proteins. It helps in relieving pain and reducing inflammation at the site of injection. Steroid injections are most commonly administered into joints, even in the small joints in your hands, to ease Arthritic pain. The number of Cortisone shots is limited because of potential side effects from the medication.

Complications include: increased pain for 24-72 hours, systemic steroid absorption, infection, and bone or tissue damage. Nerve damage, osteonecrosis (death of bone cells), tendon rupturing, and osteoporosis are other risks associated with Steroid therapy.

Steroids should not be injected if there is infection in the body or if the joint is already destroyed. In patients with bleeding problems or with anticoagulants, avoid steroid injections as it may cause bleeding at the site. Frequent steroid injections are not recommended because it increases the risk of weakening the tissues at the site of administration. It should be used no more than 3-4 times per year.

After a cortisone shot, some people may experience the feeling of warmth of the chest and face, and redness. It also increases blood sugar levels temporarily in diabetic patients. Protect the injection area after administrating a steroid injection for 2-3 days and apply ice to the injection site to relieve the pain.

b) Viscosupplementation*:* Another treatment option is Viscosupplementation and it involves thick fluid called Hyaluronic acid being injected into the joint. Hyaluronic acid is a naturally occurring substance found in joint fluid and acts as a lubricant to allow the smooth movement of bones over each other and as shock absorber for joint loads. Loss of lubrication results in joint stiffness, pain and limited movements. It is the procedure that is used in patients that are not responding to other, non-surgical methods.

The exact mechanism of action is unknown but it is proposed that injections of Hyaluronic acid temporarily restore the elastoviscosity to the synovial fluid and reduces the joint stiffness. It is also effective in reducing pain and inflammation associated with Arthritis, and may stimulate the body to produce its own Hyaluronic acid. You may experience slight swelling, pain and warmth immediately after the shot, but these symptoms are temporary.

The procedure involves aspiration of excess fluids in the case of swelling, before injecting a Hyaluronic acid injection. It is commonly used for knee arthritis.

c) Orthoses: Orthoses are the devices that are used to align the joints to function properly. There are different types of orthoses that help to maintain functions and to reduce the symptoms associated with Arthritis. Orthotic shoe inserts or well-cushioned shoes are used to reduce stress on the joints of the leg and spine. Splints that immobilize the joints result in a reduction of inflammation and pain. Braces are also used to help unstable joints. An elastic knee sleeve around the arthritic knee reduces the knee pain. These devices don't have any biochemical roles for their effects.

8) Cognitive Behavioral Therapies (CBT)

Cognitive behavioral therapy (CBT) is the form of talk therapy in which skills to identify and change negative thoughts and behaviors are developed. It says that individuals create their own experiences including pain and by changing their thoughts, awareness of pain can be changed and skills to cope with the pain are also developed. It is because the perception of pain is in your brain, therefore by addressing your thoughts and behaviors, physical pain can be reduced.

CBT provides pain relief by changing the views of people about pain and helps with coping strategies. It also changes the physical response in the brain that makes the pain worse. It makes the body's natural pain relief response more powerful by reducing the impacts of stress hormones called Serotonin & Norepinephrine in the body, thus reducing the stress and pain response. It will increase your quality of life, as pain associated with arthritis will have little interference within your daily activities.

Chapter 7) Diet & Nutrition

Diets & Nutrition for Hands & Fingers Arthritis

1) Inflammation

It is a response of the immune system to any injury, infection and irritation.

It is characterized by increased blood flow to the tissue, increased temperature, swelling, redness, and pain, which might result in dysfunction of the organ involved.

Inflammation is one of the main defense systems required by the body to recover from the infections and in the healing process of the injuries. The body responds immediately to the trauma by increasing chemicals in the body that result in heat, swelling, redness and pain. These reactions of the immune system are important in the healing process as they prevent further damage to the body by promoting pain and swelling around the injury.

Inflammation is generally of **two types**:

a. Acute inflammation

b. Chronic inflammation

In *Acute Inflammation,* the local dilation of blood vessels is involved, accompanied by vessel permeability. It is a normal, healthy, physiological process. Acute inflammation starts to occur within a few seconds or minutes after tissue injury. The damage is either physical or is caused by the immune response of the body.

Mast cells, platelets, endothelial cells and other resident cells release chemo attractants that cause leukocytes to reach at the site of injury. These cells then engulf the invading microorganisms through releasing toxins such as hydroxyl radicals, hypochlorite and superoxide radicals. Neutrophils release cytokines including interleukin (IL-1, IL-6), gamma interferon (INF-gamma), and tumor necrosis factor (TNF). Neutrophils are short lived so they are present only in the initial stages of inflammation.

a) Examples of Acute Inflammation include acute sinusitis, sore throat from flu, acute appendicitis, acute dermatitis and acute tonsillitis.

Chronic Inflammation: If the stimuli of inflammation persist then the inflammation can last for months or even years. The result of chronic inflammation could be severe damage to the body instead of the destruction of the targeted agent causing inflammation. It is mediated by long-lived macrophages and monocytes. Macrophages engulf and digest the foreign invader and release different chemical mediators that continue the pro-inflammatory response. In later stages of this process, lymphocytes invade the infected tissues, T-lymphocyte kills the infected cells and B-lymphocytes produce antibodies that destruct the invading microorganism specifically.

b) An example of Chronic Inflammation includes rheumatoid arthritis, chronic peptic ulcer, asthma, chronic sinusitis, tuberculosis, chronic active hepatitis, multiple sclerosis (MS), ulcerative colitis, and systemic lupus erythematosus (SLE).

2) Inflammation and arthritis in hands and fingers

Arthritis comes from the Latin word "arthro" that means joint, and "itis" that means inflammation. So it means inflammation of joints. People consider arthritis as a single disease but it has many forms. It may occur naturally with increase in age or it may be chronic or progressive. It may have different underlying causes; the most common are injuries and sprains. Other causes are excessive weight, joint defect or lack of physical activity. The aging process or genetic factors may also result in arthritis. The hands and fingers have multiple small joints that work together to help in motion and holding things in the hands properly. In the case of arthritis in hand and finger joints or when surrounding ligaments are inflamed, this results in pain and less mobility which results in problems dealing with routine activities.

In arthritis of hands and fingers, acute or chronic inflammation of the joints and the soft tissues surrounding it occurs, which results in trauma to the joints of hands and fingers. Degenerative arthritis mainly affects the joints of hands and other weight bearing joints. Cartilage damage in arthritis may occur because of enzyme imbalances that are released from the lining of the joint. The exact cause of this imbalance in unknown, but to repair this damage the body goes to work. It results in the growth of new bone along the sides of existing bone, which produces prominent bony lumps on the hands and fingers. The whole repair process produces severe pain in every step. In arthritis of hands and fingers, white blood cells come from the blood stream into the synovial membrane and cause the inflammation of the membrane. This inflammation results in the thickening of synovial membrane, which further releases chemicals that begin to digest bone, cartilage, tendons and ligaments of the joint. Slowly, the joint loses its shape and bones become weaker, which may lead to the loosening of joints and eventually the destruction of the joint of hands or fingers.

3) Mechanism of inflammation arthritis

Bone homeostasis is the balance between osteoblast cells (bone forming cells) and osteoclasts (bone destruction cells). In case of an inflammatory condition, inflammatory components that are mediated by the T-cells trigger the activation of osteoclast cells. It results in the destruction of bone cells at a faster rate compared to the bone formation process. It leads to bone destruction and tissue damage that further contribute to the inflammation process and destruction of the joints of bones in the hands, causing severe pain.

Lymphocytes and macrophages increase the activation of osteoclast cells through cytokines. Cytokines further promote the release of macrophage colony stimulating factors that result in increased production of macrophages and in turn osteoclast cells. The same action happens through different metabolic pathways. In the inflammation process of arthritis in hands and fingers, C-reactive protein (CRP), which is a biomarker of inflammation, has elevated serum levels. Serum levels of IL-6, TNF-alpha, IL-1 and cell adhesion molecules are also elevated during inflammation.

4) Arthritis and pain

A lot of people in our country suffer from pain. Arthritis in hands and fingers is one of the most common reasons to visit a doctor because of pain, and for using prescription drugs. In Arthritis patients, pain causes great suffering. Pain relieving drugs are never without high risks, so pain management through medicines is very disappointing as it may cause further problems. For example, COX-2 inhibitors are the new class of painkillers but it may lead to unforeseen risks and high drug costs. In Arthritis of the hands and fingers, the main cause of pain is inflammation that is caused by the immune system. So the best strategy to relieve pain is to find the cause of inflammation and remove it. Use the drugs that treat inflammation not the pain, because if inflammation stops, pain stops. More inflammation results in more pain, stiffness, swelling and loss of mobility due and therefore the patient's quality of life is affected.

5) Inflammation & Stress

Stress is significant in Arthritis as it may cause direct influence on inflammation. Nowadays, life is so busy and stressful that we can't avoid the influence of stress on our health. Sympathetic nervous system is activated when stressful events occur, which stimulates the production of the stress hormone called *Cortisol* and promotes an increase in blood sugar. Prolonged, elevated levels of cortisol may cause further problems such as thyroid dysfunction, high blood pressure, weight gain, sugar abnormalities, osteoporosis and many other metabolic imbalances.

Stress promotes inflammation through the release of certain proteins known as *neuro-peptides.* These inflammatory proteins stimulate the sympathetic nervous system and release the stress hormone i.e., Cortisol. Stress hormones further stimulate the release of acute phase proteins that are the first promoters of inflammation. The neuro-peptides that mediate stress also mediate inflammation so it is likely that stress creates the inflammatory response in the body.

High blood sugar levels that occur because of prolonged stressful situations result in increased insulin output, which leads to insulin resistance. Insulin resistance is the condition in which a high amount of blood sugar is present along with high levels of insulin, due to which insulin is not used by the insulin receptors, so it don't use blood sugar as an energy source. Prolonged high levels of insulin also trigger the production of cholesterol, so it can be stated that a continually stressful environment ultimately causes an increase in blood cholesterol levels.

Inflammation is enhanced in the presence of increased levels of interleukin-6 (IL-6), which occurs because of increased cortisol levels. Elevated levels of cortisol and IL-6 result in decreased immune activity of the body by decreasing the DHEA hormone. DHEA is an anti-aging hormone that helps in repairing and maintaining tissues, increases insulin sensitivity, reduces atherosclerosis, controls the allergic reactions and balances the immune activity of the body. So, we can say that stress exaggerates the inflammation and also decrease body's immunity, which will further worsen the arthritis. When the body deals with the stress positively it restores itself and repairs the damage caused by the stress. However, it will have a strong, negative impact if the stress builds up without any compensatory natural mechanism to counter its effects. The worsening of symptoms may lead to the worsening of the condition and results in more stress.

6) Anti-inflammatory natural food

There are many natural foods that exhibit anti-inflammatory action by enhancing anti-oxidant properties to minimize the susceptibility to the disease. Polyphenols, amino acids, alkaloids, organosulfides and terpenoids are the classes of bioactive compounds that are present in natural foods. The antioxidants present in fruits and vegetables help to control the actions of free radicals, which destroy healthy cells and exacerbate the damage at the inflamed site of injury. Sources of polyphenols in natural foods are curcumin, blueberries, grapes, peanuts, red wine and cranberries. Compounds containing terpenoids include helenalin, acanthoic acid, parthenolide, artemisinin and ursolic acid. Celastrol, panax species, pumpkins, watermelons, mushrooms and cucumbers are other examples of natural foods that have anti-inflammatory properties. Therefore, they should be used in our daily diet as they provide relief from inflammation naturally with less or no harm.

7) What is an anti-inflammation diet?

It is surprising to know that the food we eat in our daily life may cause chronic inflammation in the body and may cause arthritis in the hands and fingers. Whenever pain and inflammation related to arthritis of hands and fingers is discussed, it is always important to concentrate on diet and nutrition along with the medication as it plays a major role in causing inflammation.

The anti-inflammatory diet is based on the principle that chronic inflammation is linked with many health problems that are caused by an over-reactive immune system of the body. The anti-inflammatory diet is not a single diet that is intended for weight reduction (although it is helpful in reducing weight), nor is it an eating plan to stay on for short period of time. Rather, it is a way of preparing food lists based on scientific knowledge that can help our body in maintaining optimum health. This anti-inflammatory diet is full of whole foods; it eliminates sugars, hydrogenated oils and all other processed foods. It encourages vegetable intake for essential nutrients to ensure an energy supply to the body. Lots of fresh vegetables and fruits are the foundation of the anti-inflammatory diet. It includes one to two half-cup servings of legumes and beans, three to five half-cup servings of whole and cracked grains, and five to seven teaspoons of healthy fats every day. Bread should be avoided as it is processed and brown cooked rice is healthful. Two to six ounce servings of salmon or sardines are a good source to fulfill the daily requirement of good proteins and omega 3 fatty acids.

Other protein sources that must be avoided include natural cheese, other dairy products, omega 3 enriched eggs, and skinless meats. They can be used only three to five times per week. Water and tea can be used as beverages i.e., two to four cups of green, white or oolong tea per day are suggested. Red wine and chocolate both have anti-inflammatory properties. For sweets, sorbet, dark chocolate and unsweetened dried fruits can be used but avoid white sugar.

8) Role of the anti-inflammation diet

The Anti-inflammatory diet provides steady energy, vitamins, dietary fibers, essential fatty acids, minerals and protective phytonutrients along with influencing the inflammation of arthritis of the hands and fingers. The anti-inflammatory diet promotes easy digestion and reduces the intake of toxins, thus helping in making the body healthier. It works by supplying proper nutrients to the blood and lymph, by making food easily digestible and improving metabolism. In the body, cellular regeneration is facilitated rather than cellular degeneration that causes the disease to promote. You can start living pain free if, with medication, a diet rich in antioxidants and omega acids is used to reduce inflammation.

9) We are what we eat

Eating is not only an act of survival but also a social act that has many meanings and symbolism. All food is a source of energy. If we don't eat energy-giving foods to fuel our body then it will affect stamina and the immune system of the body, which leads to more diseases and a shorter life span. Different foods have different nutrients in them so it is necessary to have all types of food in our diet so that all necessary nutrients can be consumed. It is best to have natural foods and to avoid processed foods. Natural foods are freshly picked and have maximum vitality, which give the highest quality energy. Processed food is less natural, containing less consumable energy and more toxins. So they offer a reduced amount of nutrients compared to fresh foods. Eating in season and locally produced food is a good way to ensure vitality and quality.

How we eat and what we eat is very important. Firstly, we must choose food to eat only within the constraints of personal abilities to consume. The majority of people are overweight; that shows that our eating habits are not healthy and balanced. In arthritis, "normal" is "abnormal", which means the food that is eaten by normal individuals, very commonly including bread, pizzas, coffee etc., are not healthy for arthritis patients. Today, due to standardized foods of modern food industries, our eating is more homogenous and that is not healthy. By changing the way we eat, we can slow down the progression of many diseases, including arthritis of the hands and fingers.

10) Food allergies and intolerance

It is estimated that 2-3 tons of food is likely to be eaten by each of us in our lifetime. But when food sensitivities arise, long time favorites may be banned from our daily diet. Food sensitivity affects our lives badly as it may also involve our immune system. Food allergies are becoming common within our population, which may be due to our non-rotating diet of similar foods. In patients with food allergies, consumption of that particular food stimulates the production of antibodies that binds with the food, resulting in inflammatory response. Any inflammation in the body slows down the healing process. Furthermore, food allergens may accumulate in the body because the body does not digest them properly.

Food intolerance is the non-mediated immune response of the body that could be due to the absence of specific enzymes for metabolism. For example, enzymes needed to breakdown certain foods such as in lactose intolerance. Imbalance in microbial flora of the digestive tract could also be the reason behind food sensitivities or food intolerance. Food intolerance is more common and widespread than food allergies.

a) Food Allergy: is defined as the reaction of the body's immune system to food or any food ingredient that is considered as foreign by the body.

b) Food Intolerance: It is an adverse reaction to food ingredients or any additive in food, but it does not involve the immune system and usually involves the digestive system only.

c) Food Sensitivity: It includes both food intolerance and food allergy.

d) Food hypersensitivity is of two types: *Allergic food hypersensitivity & Non-allergic food hypersensitivity.*

Allergic food hypersensitivity has a further two types: *IgE-mediated food allergy & Non-IgE-mediated food allergy.*

e) The difference between Food Allergy and Non-allergic FHS is that *Food allergy* is caused by one or more food proteins interacting with the immune system of the body. And *Non-allergic food hypersensitivity* occurs because of any substance other than the food proteins and it doesn't involve the immune system of the body.

The frequency of food sensitivities has increased in the last few decades. This is explained by some of the factors including hygiene theory, pollution, modern agricultural methods, skin testing for allergies, and intestinal well-being.

11) Food allergy symptoms

Adverse effects that occur due to food allergies could be of many types and may involve many areas of the body. The most common site that is affected due to food allergy is the digestive tract. Other target areas include skin and mucous membranes, the nervous system, respiratory tract, and muscles.

a) Symptoms of food allergy are Nausea, Vomiting, Diarrhea, Indigestion, Belching, Constipation, Abdominal pain, Eczema, Redness, Itching, Swelling, Sneezing, Runny nose, Asthma, Chest constriction, Lung spasms, Coughing, Muscle ache, Watery eyes, Migraine, Dizziness, Headaches, Hyperactivity, Irritability, Lack of concentration, Depression.

b) Severity of symptoms of allergy ranges from mild to severe depending on the body's response. The situation may get worse if symptoms of more than one allergy are present, affecting different target areas. For example, inflammation in the digestive system due to infection may help other microorganisms to get into the system. In a stressful environment, the symptoms of food allergies may appear to be worse. Symptoms of a food allergy may appear after minutes, hours, or days after food ingestion.

12) Food allergy diagnosis

Different phony tests are available for diagnosis of food allergies in arthritis of the hands and fingers. But the desire for simple and confirmatory tests for diagnosis of a food allergy is very simple to understand but it is not practical. It is because the process of food allergy is very complex and may involve so many variables affecting the process. No single test can show the complex nature of this reaction. No tricks and short cuts are available for that, so if anyone claims to diagnose the food allergy with any test then he is making a false claim. There are no valid definitive tests for the diagnosis of food allergies that cause arthritis in the hands and fingers and the only way to improve this condition is to revise the dieting habits. "Vega meters" and "Muscle tests" are performed by the physicians for diagnosis but they are not definitive tests for food allergies.

The key to diet revision success is to remove the food antigen; mostly food proteins that are responsible for causing or contributing to the arthritis. Other important goals for diet revision are to change your lifestyle to support a new diet plan, to achieve optimal nutrition and to achieve appropriate weight.

13) Food sensitivity and arthritis

The role of food sensitivity in arthritis in the hands and fingers is often neglected due to many reasons that include different forms of arthritis having different rates of occurrence in different individuals and multiple origins. Secondly, the adverse reactions are more delayed in food intolerance than in patients with a true allergy. Thirdly, symptoms of food sensitivity are triggered by different lifestyle factors, such as smoking, food intake, exercise, medications and intestinal infections. Fourthly, the reactions of food sensitivity are different for different foods in different individuals. Thus, no single dietary change will help in improving your food allergy symptoms. However, many researchers have shown that the severity of arthritis of hands and fingers, its pain and inflammation, is diminished in people when they undergo a supervised fast. So there is a great need of detailed and well-designed studies to understand the role of diet in the treatment of arthritis of all kinds.

Food that triggers food sensitivity include food dyes especially red and yellow, chocolate containing caffeine, dried fruits due to their concentrated sugars, onions, some vinegars, bananas, aspartame, meat preservatives, monosodium glutamate (MSG) and pickled herring. This diet removes the major food allergens, but if someone experiences food allergy symptoms even after following the diet closely then removal of all other potential irritants is recommended from the diet.

14) Foods that cause & increase inflammation

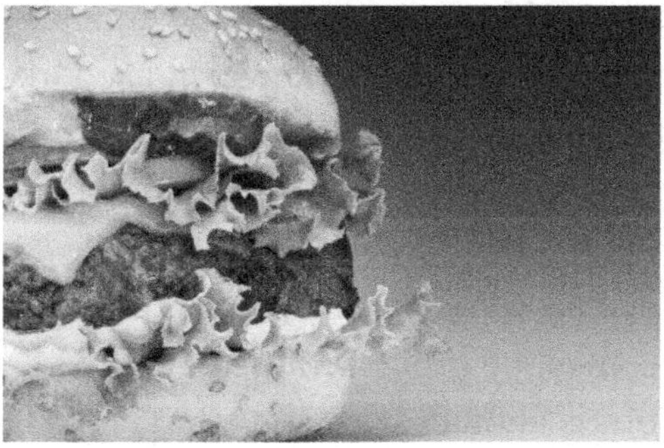

Certain changes in the diet are helpful in reducing pain and inflammation in various types of arthritis. If it is known that a certain type of food is linked with specific food allergy symptoms then it is wise to avoid those foods.

Increased symptoms of allergy have been linked with wheat and gluten, dairy products and other animal products, refined sugar, yeast, soy, citrus fruits, and nightshade vegetables (e.g., bell peppers, tomatoes, eggplant, potatoes, hot peppers and tobacco are in this family). Sugars must be avoided as it may cause many abnormal reactions. It depresses the immune system of the body. Wheat is also the major cause of food allergy as it is the most frequently consumed grain in our daily lives. Today, wheat is not what it was hundreds of years ago as it is genetically modified now and contains a maximum gluten percentage in it. Gluten is the protein that reacts with the immune system pathologically and produces inflammation. Citrus fruits may exaggerate arthritis in hands and fingers as they cause inflammation. Alcohol should be avoided as it is turned into sugar in the body and may depress the immune system. Dairy products are also a very important and common trigger of food allergy as it contains high fats. High contents of fat-soluble toxins that are stored in the body are the primary allergens. Other than that, toxins present in the animal feed in the form of pesticide residues are very dangerous. Dairy products put lots of toxins into the body's immune system due to the presence of hormones and steroids in the diets of the animals. So these dairy products must be avoided. Commercial eggs, pork and beef should be avoided because of the acidifying nature and toxin contents of the animal proteins. Beef and pork are rich in arachidonic acid, which promotes inflammation. Peanuts and shellfish should also be avoided as aflatoxins are grown on the surface of peanuts, so peanuts must be processed to avoid the production of such toxins. Corn is another common allergen that should be avoided because of a heavy bombardment of pesticides. It is unlikely for an individual to have all of these triggers so if someone is willing to try this approach, he/she has to eliminate particular foods from the above list at one time to observe if symptoms persist or not. When we stop taking reactive food that triggers the food allergy, we may undergo a period of withdrawal.

But within seven to ten days of eliminating trigger foods from our diet, positive changes may occur.

15) Anti-inflammation diet

The anti-inflammatory diet is very important in managing arthritis in the hands and fingers through food. Our body needs all types of nutrients that are present in different natural foods. So to get that fuel for our body we need to eat natural and fresh foods, not the canned processed foods. The vital micronutrients such as vitamins, minerals and phyto-chemicals can be obtained through supplementation to support the metabolic system of the body and for energy needs. However, macronutrients including proteins, carbohydrates and fats that are needed for body's fuel can come only from fresh food. The anti-inflammatory diet also helps in reducing weight as it contains moderate-calories. But don't restrict your calorie intake if you are eating the right food.

16) Macro Nutrients

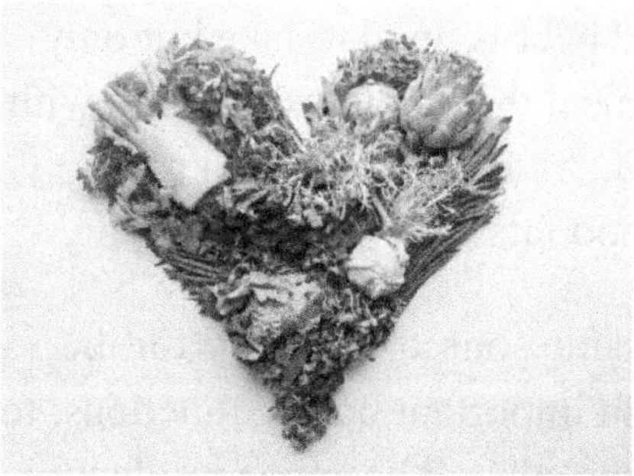

All of us need energy to do our daily activities and to live healthily, and we get energy from food we eat daily. Basic constituents of food include carbohydrates, fats and proteins. These are called macronutrients as they are greatly used by the body as the source of energy and they are the major part of our diet. In the anti-inflammatory diet, macronutrients play a very important role in reducing inflammation of arthritis of the hands and fingers. Among nutrients, only carbohydrates, fats and proteins contain calories.

a) Proteins: They are required for growth and function, tissue replacement, maintenance, in hormone and enzyme growth and production, and in the production of antibodies. Proteins are made up of Amino-acids and Amino acids are further **classed** as *essential amino acids*, *non-essential amino acids*, *conditionally essential*, and *other that are not found in body proteins.*

The adult protein intake should be 45-60 grams per day as eating enough good-quality protein at each meal is the best way to maintain the body's energy levels. Organic sources for proteins are the best choice in order to avoid antibiotics, pesticide residues and hormones. **Dietary sources for proteins are:** meat, fish, eggs, dairy, soybean, oats, chocolate, walnut, wheat, asparagus, raw spinach, cabbage, seeds, rye, legumes, cod, chickpeas, and avocados.

For meat eaters, organic, grass fed beef is good to take but only one to two servings per week. A meal that contains legumes with grains is the best source of protein. Avocado contains a good amount of proteins, along with good fats.

b) Fats: Lipids or fats are the usable source of energy for the body. Fats are required to maintain important bodily functions, to build cell membranes, for tissue growth and hormone production and for the formation of leukotriene and prostaglandins that are the regulators of the inflammatory process. We need to concentrate more on the type of fats we take rather than on the amount of fats. Fats are composed of fatty acids and fatty acids are of two **types**: *Essential fatty acids* and *Non-essential fatty acids*.

Types of fats are *saturated fats*, *unsaturated fats*, *monounsaturated fats* and *polyunsaturated fats*.

Saturated fats are normally present in dairy products, poultry, red meat, in palm oil and coconut oil. They are required in our diet to produce cholesterol in the body, which is a precursor of many important hormones (for example cortisol, progesterone, and aldosterone) and is also the important component of the cell membrane. They are solid fat at room temperature. Examples of saturated fats are butter, palm oil and coconut oils. They are considered dangerous.

Unsaturated fats are liquid forms of fats at room temperature. Vegetable oil is an example of unsaturated fats.

Monounsaturated fats contain one double bond between carbon atoms. Olive oil, canola oil and fats present in avocados contain this. They are also called "good fats" and taking a sufficient amount of monounsaturated fats helps in decreasing LDL cholesterol, which is a "bad fat".

Polyunsaturated fats contain two or more double bonds between carbon atoms. They are made up of omega fatty acids and are less stable than saturated fats. Vegetable oils are the example of polyunsaturated fats. Omega 3 fatty acids can be used 3-4 times per week.

Hydrogenated oils stimulate inflammation promoting prostaglandins, thus promoting the inflammation process. They are chemically modified from room temperature liquid state to solid state and contain trans-fatty acids.

Carbohydrates: Building blocks of carbohydrates are monosaccharides. Unprocessed and unrefined carbohydrates are a good energy source. Legumes, whole wheat, barley, fresh vegetables, whole oats, sweet potatoes and brown rice are the good **source of complex carbohydrates**. Simple carbohydrates that are present in processed, sweetened foods should be excluded or limited from the diet. The **sources of simple carbohydrates** include fruits, pastries, white flour, soda pop, white rice, sugar, caffeinated beverages, and cereals made with enriched grains or sugar content or other products containing "wheat" or "whole wheat".

Increased levels of sugar cause an increase in insulin production and triggers cholesterol synthesis. So it can be said that simple carbohydrates containing products cause high cholesterol, obesity, and diabetes and also cause an increase in inflammation of arthritis. Foods containing a high percentage of carbohydrates increase the inflammatory markers and processed foods with less glycemic content may modulate the effects of inflammation.

c) Fiber: It helps in giving bulk to the stool so that it can pass through the intestine easily. It also helps in ensuring that toxins aren't absorbed from the tract into the blood stream as it increases the transient time. 40-50 g of fiber per day is good to include in our daily diet. Dietary fiber is of two **types**: Soluble Fiber & Insoluble Fiber.

Soluble Fiber helps in reducing blood sugar levels and also blood cholesterol levels. It can be further sub-categorized as: Hemicellulose, pectin, mucilage and gum. **Sources** of Soluble fiber are psyllium seed husks, nuts, oats, barley, rye, legumes, fruits including avocados, plums, berries, and ripe bananas, vegetables including carrots and broccoli.

Insoluble Fiber softens the stool and the best example of insoluble fiber is wheat bran containing a high amount of cellulose. **Sources** of insoluble fiber are potato skin, beans, peas, whole grain foods, lignans, cauliflowers, and the skin of grapes, and tomatoes.

17) Making Choices

A busy urban life and hectic work schedule are primarily responsible for the failure to eat regular meals. Furthermore, busy work habits and home activities prevent the caloric intake from being distributed evenly throughout the day. One of the worst habits is to eat dinner very late, and then to sleep immediately after that without allowing the complete digestion of the food. We are often sleeping when we should be digesting food we just ate, and it is known that during sleep the metabolic process is slow.

Furthermore, in our children there is great need for energy yielding foods that promote good health and growth. It is the duty of the parents to set the example for children about dieting habits, and make them aware of the importance of a healthy and balanced diet. People who understand the importance of a balanced, healthy diet can teach the rest of the population about the important nutrients that promote health and help in fighting diseases. Poor lifestyle choices including lack of exercise and smoking contribute to different diseases including risk of infection. Infections can further complicate the situation that might result in exaggerated arthritis of the hands and fingers. Avoid using painkillers, as addressing the cause is more logical rather than masking the symptoms.

A healthy diet containing lots of fresh fruits, vegetables, fish, olive oils, and other supportive food may help us to live a healthy life, as well as to avoid painkillers so that the side effects of these medications can be eliminated.

18) Recommended meal times

A proper; healthy diet is our best friend in the battle against symptoms of arthritis in the hands and fingers. It is best to eat healthy food at regularly scheduled times of the day. How often we eat is also very important in maintaining our health. In managing arthritis of the hands and fingers, the standard three times a day meal is not ideal, rather it is good to eat four to five times a day in small amounts. Eating daily at the same time will help to establish a pattern with the endocrine system of the body, resulting in facilitated digestion at those particular times. Make sure to eat breakfast daily with whole grains as it helps in reducing the risk of insulin resistance. Eating all meals at proper times throughout the day is very important in maintaining a good metabolic rate of the body. Avoid eating late at night because the metabolism is at its slowest at that time.

Properly chewing the food ingested is very important and this should be practiced during each meal. If food is not chewed thoroughly then digestion will be improper, which will result in less absorption of important nutrients from the food. After thorough chewing of the ingested food, the nearly liquefied product will enter the stomach and absorption is much easier.

Don't eat food randomly anytime in the day, that means avoid eating while watching television or talking on the phone. Have a relaxed and quite environment while eating so that you can enjoy it. Do not drink high volumes of liquids while eating, and if it is necessary to take any liquid then take it in small sips.

19) Suggestions to follow

Anti-inflammatory and circulation boosting spices such as turmeric, ginger and cinnamon should be used liberally in cooking. Make carrot and ginger soup, use turmeric while stirring fries, and use ginger and cinnamon spiced pears. Delicious and healing!

Include carbohydrates, proteins and fats in each meal so that the energy needs of the body can be fulfilled. Use extra-virgin olive oil in main cooking. Furthermore, in grocery stores read labels of items and avoid anything that is hydrogenated or partially hydrogenated. All types of fruits, especially berries, and all vegetables, especially beans, along with whole grains should be the part of a routine diet as they are rich in fiber and provide the daily required phyto-nutrients. Avoid crash dieting or fasting and increase dietary calcium to reduce the risk of osteoporosis in later years of life.

Metabolic wastes are stored primarily in the connective tissues of the body. When antibiotics and other anti-inflammatory drugs are used regularly, the excess toxins of these drugs are stored in tissues that will eventually interfere with the weak immune system, or weak organs of the body. Drinking plenty of water, fresh air and exercise flushes out these stored toxins. Avoid alcoholic drinks.

20) Daily diet plans

The main nutrition principles in the treatment of arthritis of hands and fingers are to eat sensibly and healthily and to reduce your weight. Include sources of omega 3 fatty acids in the diet. The meal plan is designed according to the average individual's needs to help him/her lose weight. It is a nutritionally balanced plan but food choices may vary according to more individual lifestyles, nutritional requirements and daily routines. Use this diet plan to have an idea to create your own diet plan and drink plenty of water throughout your day.

21) Diet plan for osteo arthritis

At ***breakfast*** drink 200ml fruit juice, or amug of weak tea, and eat porridge 30g with 150 ml skimmed milk, 200-300mg chondroitin supplement + 500-1000mg glucosamine.

At ***mid-morning*** eat some fruits and have water.

At ***lunch*** eat a mixed salad with a sandwich that comprises of granary bread, a thin slice of chicken or hem with olive oil-based spread. Drink plenty of water and a low sugar, low fat yoghurt, and 200-300mg chondroitin supplement + 500-1000mg glucosamine.

At ***nid-afternoon***, eat fruits and drink water.

For your ***evening meal*** eat whole-wheat pasta 40g or basmati rice 40g or a small chicken breast or a small portion of lean meat or 2-3 small potatoes, with loads of vegetables, fruits and water. Also take 200-300mg chondroitin supplement + 500-1000mg glucosamine.

In the ***evening*** eat fruit, 1-2 oatcakes, and drink water.

22) Diet plan for rheumatoid arthritis

For ***Breakfast*** eat 125ml cooked porridge (oats), 200ml apple juice, three fish fingers on one slice of whole wheat toast with canola margarine.

As a ***light meal*** eat 125ml tossed salad that contains 1 cucumber, a small tomato and lettuce with low fat salad dressing. Eat a cheddar cheese and ham sandwich containing 30 g ham and 30 g cheese with 2 slices of whole bread with canola margarine.

As a ***Main meal*** eat 125ml brown rice, 125ml butternut, 120g chicken, 50 ml sauce of your choice, 125ml of cauliflower with 1 cup of fruit salad.

Chapter 8) Exercises and Alternative Treatments

Exercises and Alternative Treatments for Arthritis in the Hands & Fingers

1) Exercises

A joint needs lubrication for easy and smooth movement of the bones, which makes the joint just like a moving part of any machine or engine that needs oil. As we discussed in earlier chapters, the ends of a bone are covered with smooth cartilage to make gliding of one bone over another easier. The lining of this joint capsule is called synovial membrane and is very thin in normal joints with a few blood vessels. Normal joints move easily without any pain but if there is any abnormality in the joint then it will cause pain and inflammation during movement. In an inflamed joint, this lining of the joint capsule is very thick with many white blood cells that produce chemicals that cause inflammation. Suppression of this inflammation to prevent long-term joint damage is the main goal in arthritis of hands and fingers.

One proven method to reduce inflammation is regular and gentle exercise. Movement puts pressure on the cartilage and joint to help synovial fluid to oil the joint through improved circulation. People usually hesitate to move the painful joint but it is not a healthy option as it will damage the joint even further and will result in muscle weakness, tightness, stiffness and freezing of the joint. Exercise doesn't mean to hurt anyone or to exaggerate one's pain, but physical pain can be avoided if exercise is done within the limits of your ease and ability.

Some people are not interested in regular, formal exercise activities but they prefer to perform daily activities such as gardening, light housework, clearing walks and driveways, leisure walking or exercises in a pool. These activities also have health benefits. Exercise doesn't need to be continuous; rather it can be divided into three to four 10-minute sessions per day. Exercising with moderate intensity has shown best results in studies but it should be practiced regularly. Otherwise, exercising twice a week will yield no results.

2) The Benefits of Exercise

It helps to improve balance and have a better sense of control, provides better quality of sleep, regulates breathing patterns and body temperature, and boosts self-confidence and also helps in reducing other health problems. In people with Arthritis of the hands and fingers, exercise is very crucial, because when arthritis immobilizes you, only exercise can make you move on. Exercise helps in reducing joint pain and fatigue, and in increasing strength and flexibility of muscles. It also helps to maintain bone strength, controls body weight and makes you feel better by giving more strength and energy to get you through the day.

3) Preparation for Exercise

a) Consult your doctor: Talk to your doctor about the types of exercises possible according to the severity of disease and joints involved. Discuss with him about the specific movements that should be avoided or specific exercises that should be adopted to aid your pain management. Stiffness, pain and fatigue are the main barriers to exercise success in patients with arthritis of hands and fingers. But preparing for exercise after discussing all the issues with your doctor or the physical therapist will either eliminate or reduce these issues.

b) Warm up: The Purpose of Warm-up is to increase the temperature of muscles and joints and to improve the circulation so that the body becomes comfortable, easily moveable, and less stiff with decreased risk of injury. At the end of the warm-up procedure, your body will feel slightly warmer and the recommended time for warm-up in patients with arthritis of hands and fingers is 12-14 minutes. Warm-up activities may include: flexibility exercises, marching, walking or biking at a half normal speed.

c) Cool down: The purpose of this phase is to return your heart rate to a few beats above normal. This helps to prevent dizziness, a sudden drop in blood pressure, fainting and the feeling of nausea.

4) Exercise Program

You need your hands in all activities such as in cooking, cleaning, typing, brushing your teeth, buttoning your shirt and opening a jar, or anything else. You don't understand the importance of the involvement of your hands in your routine life until you suffer from Arthritis of the hands and fingers. Regular physical activity has shown to decrease the inflammation markers so exercise is very important in pain management and reducing the severity of arthritis in the hands and fingers. Try to improve your range of motion so that you can perform your daily tasks more easily.

The *three types of exercises* that help in the fitness program and in managing arthritis of hands and fingers are:

5) Range of movement or Stretching Exercises

They help to reduce stiffness, improve flexibility and strength and promote good posture. It involves movement of joints through their normal range, for example rolling your shoulders backward and forward, and raising your arms over your head. Stretching exercises can be done daily or every other day and include: golf, t'ai chi and swimming.

a) Strengthening Exercises: These exercises make hand and wrist muscles strong. Strengthening exercises also provide protection to the joints. Weight training is an example. Strengthening exercises should be done every other day.

b) Aerobics Exercises or Endurance Exercises: These exercises help in the overall fitness of the body by raising your heartbeat and improving your level of fitness by strengthening your cardiovascular system. It also controls your weight and gives you better stamina. Give 20-30 minutes to the aerobic exercises three times a week, or you can split the time into 10-minute blocks for your ease. Examples include: brisk walking, tennis, cycling and riding a bike.

6) Distinction between OA & RA Exercises:

The distinction between hand pain induced due to OA and RA is very important for many reasons. If the pain in the hand is induced due to RA then don't alleviate it with exercise alone because disease modifying anti-rheumatic drugs (DMARDs) have shown to slow the disease progression and also limit the joint damage, reducing the chances that your hand will become permanently disfigured. Then you should perform any type of exercise with caution to avoid any further damage to the joints of hand. Thirdly, strengthening exercises can be harmful if they are performed aggressively, so patients with rheumatoid arthritis in the hands and fingers should perform exercises moderately. The main issue is, whether people have RA or OA, they should respect the pain and perform exercises gently to avoid further harm to your joints.

7) Exercising with Osteoarthritis:

Some *tips for exercising with osteoarthritis* include:

Do exercise regularly to reduce the symptoms of arthritis of hands and fingers. Muscles surrounding joints will be stronger if you exercise regularly and actively, resulting in decreased joint deterioration. It will also help in weight reduction, as it will put less strain on your joints. The most important thing is to exercise gently rather than aggressively because it will further cause pain and joint deterioration and never force or exert pressure on a painful joint. Instead, try to do small exercises in divided sessions to improve the range of movement and stamina of the body.

8) Exercises with rheumatoid arthritis

Some *tips for exercising with rheumatoid arthritis* include:

The most important tip is to have a balance between the session of rest and activity in patients with rheumatoid arthritis of the hands. The intensity of the workout should be reduced and you should exercise when you are least tired; try to do small exercises every day so that your range of movements is improved. Strengthening exercises help in building muscles and also help to support and protect your joints. Exercising in the morning time will help you in reducing morning stiffness and will give you energy for the whole day. Maintenance of good posture at all times is very important in rheumatoid arthritis patients; cycling, swimming, and brisk walking are good for people with rheumatoid arthritis.

Rheumatoid arthritic patients should not perform exercise of squeezing balls, for example, as it puts more stress on the joints.

The most important rule for arthritic patients is that hand exercises for rheumatoid arthritis should not hurt, if you are experiencing pain then stop the hand exercise immediately. When the pain subsides, you can continue with your exercises but with reduced intensity. After performing a hand exercise with low intensity, if the pain comes back, consult your doctor as it may be something more than arthritis.

9) Hand Exercises in Arthritis in the Hands & Fingers

a) Finger Joint Blocking:

Put your hand on the table, palm down and with the opposite hand hold the affected finger at the middle just below where the joint ends. First bend the finger then straighten it at the end of the joint, keep all other fingers straight. Then repeat it for each finger of the hand.

b) Wrist Bend: Bend your wrist forward and then backward with your arm outstretched.

c) Wrist Turn: With an outstretched arm, turn the palm of your hand upwards to face the ceiling and then downwards to face the floor.

d) Muscle Strengthener 1: Hold a piece of newspaper or any other paper by the corner with your hand, and then crumble it into a ball as fast as possible by using only one hand.

e) Muscle Strengthener 2: Put your hand on the table palm facing downwards, and then place your other hand on the top of that hand. Lift up your hand using the fingers of the hand on the bottom; it can be done by lifting all fingers at once or one at a time.

f) Thumb Stretch: Outstretch your hand and then bend your thumb towards the base of the little finger, then return the thumb back to the original position, and repeat it many times.

g) Finger Curls: Outstretch your hand, keeping your wrist straight, extend and spread your fingers. Then make a fist with your hand, keeping the thumb on the outer side of the fingers. Make sure that you make a loose fist and don't squeeze it tightly.

h) Finger to Palm: Hold your wrist upright and straight with straight fingers. Bend your small finger slowly towards palm of the hand and hold the position for 5-10 seconds. Relax your hand by bringing your little finger back to normal position. Repeat it with rest of your fingers and do it twice daily.

i) Finger touch: With an open hand touch your thumb to the pad just below the little finger. Release and then touch the tips of your pointer finger, middle finger, ring finger and little finger with your thumb in sequence.

j) Bending Fingers: Gently straighten your fingers and keep them close-by. Then make a curve with your fingers by bending only the middle and end joints of the fingers but keeping your knuckles and wrist straight. Return to the original position by moving your joints slowly and smoothly, repeat this exercise with your other hand and do it many times.

k) Bending Knuckles: Stretch out your hands, keeping the fingers closed. Bend the knuckles of your hand keeping the finger joints straight and hold the position for 10 seconds. Return back to the original position by moving your fingers and repeat this exercise twice.

l) Stretch to fist: Have your hand straight with your fingers straight and close together. Slowly spread the fingers and then make a fist. Hold your hand in this position for 5 seconds and repeat this exercise twice per day.

m) Stretching fingers: Put your hand on the table, palm down and spread and stretch your fingers wide apart. Then relax your fingers slowly by bringing them together. Again stretch your fingers and repeat it many times with the other hand also.

n) The OK: Have your hand with fingers, wrist and thumb upwards and make an O shape by touching the tip of your index finger with the tip of your thumb. Hold thc position for at least 10-15 seconds and repeat it 5-10 times. Do this exercise twice per day.

o) Finger Walking: Place your hand on the table with the palm facing down and fingers spread apart. Lift and move your index finger slowly towards the thumb without changing the position of the thumb. Then slowly lift and move the middle finger towards the thumb as done before. Repeat it with all other fingers one by one and then with other hand. Do not move your thumb or wrist as your fingers walk towards the thumb.

10) Hand Exercises for Rheumatoid Arthritis

a) Hand Exercise No.1: Have your hand upright with your fingers, thumb and wrist pointing upward. Hold it for 5 to 10 seconds.

b) Hand Exercise No.2: Keep your hand in an upward position, with your wrist straight. Then bend the base joints of the fingers connecting the fingers to the palm, keeping your middle and end joints straight. Hold twice per day with each hand.

c) Hand Exercise No.3: Outstretch your hand with straight knuckles and fingers spread slowly like an opening up fan. Then from this position make a fist and hold each position for 5 seconds. Repeat on both hands twice per day.

d) Hand Exercise No.4: Bend each of your fingers downwards from the base joint using your other hand to bend your fingers. Then bend your finger using second row of the knuckles in your finger and repeat it using third row of joints that is closest to the fingertips. Hold for 10 seconds and repeat for all the 10 fingers twice a day.

e) Hand Exercise No.5: Keep your hand and fingers straight, pointing upwards and bend your fingers downwards to touch the palm of your hand. Only touch the palm of your hand with your fingers and don't make a fist. Hold for 5 seconds and repeat on both hands twice per day.

f) Hand Exercise No.6: With your fingers, thumb and wrist pointing upward, make an "O" by touching the tip of the index finger to the tip of your thumb. Hold it for 10-20 seconds and repeat on both hands 2-10 times twice per day.

g) Hand Exercise No.7: Keep your wrist and base joints straight, bending only the middle and end joints of the finger towards the palm of your hand and hold each position for 5 seconds. Repeat it on all ten fingers twice per day.

These hand exercises are effective for maintaining mobility in your hands and stretching if you have RA. These exercises are not for strength because strength comes with good hand mobility and is enough for doing daily living activities.

11) Hand exercises for Osteo Arthritis

a) Finger Lift: Put your hand on the table with the palm facing down and gently lift one of your fingers and then lower it back. Repeat it with all the fingers and thumb one by one or you can also try it all at the same time. Repeat it 10-12 times on both hands. It will increase flexibility in your fingers.

b) Make A Fist: Hand and finger exercises help in relieving pain by strengthening your hands and fingers and also in increasing the range of motion. Stretch your hand until it is comfortable for you and you don't feel pain. Then gently wrap your thumb across your fingers and make a fist. Hold it for 45 to 60 seconds then relax your hand and spread your fingers wide. Repeat with both hands at least four times.

c) Claw Stretch: Hold your hand in front of you so that your palm is facing you, bend your fingertips downwards so that they can touch the base of each finger joint, making a claw like shape. Hold in this position for 45 to 60 seconds and then relax your hand. Repeat this exercise on each hand four times per day. This exercise will improve the range of motion in your hands.

d) Finger Stretch: Put your hand on the table with the palm facing down and straighten your fingers gently without forcing your joints. This will help in pain relief and will improve the range of motion of your hands and fingers. Hold it for 45-60 seconds and then relax your hand. Repeat with both hands, 4 times per day.

e) Grip Strengthener: Hold a small, soft ball in your palm and squeeze it as forcefully as you can. Hold for a few seconds and then release. Repeat it 10 to 15 times on both hands, two to three times per week. Make sure that you have a rest period of 48 hours between the sessions. Don't perform this exercise if the thumb joint is damaged. This exercise will help in opening doorknobs and holding things without dropping them easily.

f) Pinch Strengthener: Pinch a soft foam ball with the tips of the fingers and thumb and hold it for 30-60 seconds. Repeat on both hands 10-15 times, two to three times per week. Make sure to give your hands a rest of at least 48 hours and don't exercise if the thumb joint of your hand is damaged. This exercise will result in strong muscles of your fingers and thumb as you can open food packages, turn keys and use a pump more easily.

g) Thumb Extension: Put your hand on the table and wrap a rubber band around your fingers at the base of the finger joints. Then gently move your thumb away from all the fingers as far as you can easily do and hold for 45-60 seconds, and then relax your hand. Repeat this on both hands 10-15 times, two to three times per week, giving a rest period of 48 hours to the hands. It will result in strong thumb muscles so that you can grab bottles and cans easily.

h) Thumb Flax: Outstretch your hand with the palm facing upwards. Then extend your thumb away from the fingers as far as you can, then bend your thumb across your palm so that it touches the base of your small finger. Hold this for 45-60 seconds and repeat with both the thumbs four times.

i) Thumb Stretches: With your hands straight, palm facing you, gently bend the tip of your thumb towards the base of your index finger. Hold it for 45-60 seconds and then relax your hand. Repeat it four times. Then gently stretch your thumb across your palm with your lower thumb joint. Hold it for 45-60 seconds and then relax your hand. Repeat it four times again.

j) Thumb Touch: With your hand in front of you, having a straight wrist, gently touch the tip of your thumb with each of your fingertips one by one making an "O". Hold each position for 45-60 seconds and repeat on each hand four times. This exercise will help in picking up your toothbrush, pens when you write, a fork and spoon and other things like that.

12) Tips for Arthritic Fingers

If your hands and fingers are painful and stiff then warm up by moving and stretching your fingers. You can use a heating pad or also soak them in warm water for about 5-10 minutes. Rubbing oil on your hands can also be carried out for deeper warmth. Rubber gloves or soaking hands in warm water for a few minutes also helps.

Playing with clay is one of the best ways to increase the range of motion, and to strengthen your hands. You can also try squishing the clay into balls with your palms or use your fingertips to roll it into snakes, or to pinch spikes on a dinosaur.

Activities such as playing the piano or knitting can keep your fingers alert and can reduce the pain associated with arthritis of hands and fingers. Other activities could be typing or cutting the vegetables for soup.

Add accessories to the knobs of the doors for easy turning and use lightweight household pans, pots and utensils. Use lightweight plastic dishes and cups and replace drinking glasses with stemware. Try a shoehorn with long handles to put your shoes without any stress of bending over and stretching your hands.

13) Home Remedies & Alternative Treatments

Arthritis of the hands and fingers causes discomfort and uneasiness, as we use our hands and fingers for doing most of our daily activities. Thanks to medical advances, there are many methods for reducing symptoms of arthritis. So along with medications, highly effective and natural home remedies can also be used to improve the condition of your hands and fingers.

The most important *Home Remedies used for Arthritis of hands and fingers* are:

a) **Honey and Cinnamon:** This combination has excellent healing properties as honey has antiseptic qualities and cinnamon has antioxidant and antimicrobial properties. This mixture helps in reducing muscle stiffness and in relaxing the body. Mix half a teaspoon of cinnamon powder and one tablespoon of honey on a daily basis and take it every morning on an empty stomach.

b) Olive Oil: There is a special compound known as *oleocanthal* present in olive oil that helps in preventing the production of pro-inflammatory COX-1 and COX-2 enzymes. It helps in reducing inflammation and pain associated with arthritis of the hands and fingers. Olive oil is used in cooking but it can also be used to massage your hands and fingers.

c) Potatoes: Potatoes have anti-inflammatory and anti-oxidant properties that help in treating hand arthritis. Potato juice can be prepared by cutting a medium-sized potato into slices without peeling the skin. Then put the slices in cold water overnight. Strain the solution the next morning and drink the water on an empty stomach daily, it will relieve the pain of the joints and make joints more flexible.

d) Alfalfa Seeds*:* Tea made from alfalfa seeds has beneficial results in treating arthritis of the hands. To make tea, add one teaspoon of seeds to one cup of boiling water. Take 3-4 cups of tea daily for two weeks to reduce inflammation. Another option is to take Alfalfa capsules or add small a amount of alfalfa to your diet.

e) Castor Oil **:**It has powerful curative and medicinal properties as *Ricinoleic acid* present in Castor oil has analgesic, anti-bacterial and anti-inflammatory functions. So it is very effective in relieving arthritis pain. You can massage it gently into the affected area twice daily to reduce pain. Another option is to boil two tablespoons of Castor oil and then add it into fresh orange juice. Take this glass of juice before eating your breakfast daily to notice improvement in your condition.

f) Apple Cider Vinegar*:* It helps in reducing pain and stiffness in arthritic hands as it has anti-inflammatory and alkalizing properties. Take a glass of warm water mixed with one tablespoon of apple cider vinegar and some honey daily. Warming the apple cider vinegar with a small amount of cayenne pepper to make a paste and then applying this warm paste to painful joints will give you relief from the stiffness, soreness and pain of arthritis.

g) Turmeric*:* It is a popular ingredient that can be used in hand arthritis due to its anti-inflammatory properties. Turmeric also has antibacterial and antiseptic properties that help in killing the bacteria as well as giving protection to the infected finger from an attack from microorganisms. Mix a teaspoon of turmeric with warm milk along with honey and drink it to get relief from the symptoms of arthritis. Another option is to make a paste by adding a few drops of mustard oil to one teaspoon of turmeric powder, mixing it properly to make thick paste. Apply the paste to swollen fingers and leave it for half an hour, then wash the area with lukewarm water. This will also help in reducing pain and inflammation.

h) Garlic*:* It is another effective ingredient that contains anti-inflammatory properties and can be used in the treatment of arthritic hands and fingers. It helps in reducing the pain and inflammation associated with arthritis. Garlic contains *Allicin,* which helps the body to suppress the reproduction of microorganisms that worsen the symptoms. Eat garlic on a regular basis either in raw or cooked form. Or you may massage the oil that is made after heating garlic cloves in mustard oil. Repeat it many times a day to get easy and quick relief.

To conclude, you also need to follow the doctor's advice along with these home remedies for hand arthritis. Never neglect exercises and physical therapies to have better joint movements of your hands and fingers.

14) Alternative Therapies

People use alternative treatment therapies because they have persistent pain, their symptoms are not effectively controlled by conventional therapy, they are concerned about the side effects of conventional medications or they want to use natural treatment. Some of the most commonly used alternative therapies used for arthritis of hands and fingers include:

a) **T'ai chi***:* T'ai chi is one of the methods used for pain reduction in arthritic patients. The movements of Tai chi are graceful and gentle, making this practice suitable for patients of arthritis of the hands and fingers. It helps in increasing the range of motion of the muscles in hands and fingers and also strengthens the joints. It also encourages the mind to focus away from pain. It involves many movements that are performed at a slow speed, accompanied by deep breathing. Don't use this therapy without consulting a doctor as certain postures might be contraindicated in Arthritic patients. T'ai chi helps in decreasing stress and also helps in increasing the flexibility of the muscles and enhances the immune system of the body.

b) Massage*:* Massage is a general term used for manipulating skin muscles, tendons and ligaments, rubbing and pressing them. Massage therapists use their hands and fingers, sometimes forearms, elbows or even feet for the massage. Massages can be done with varying pressure and movements according to the requirement and may range from light stroking to deep pressure. A massage therapy session involves different types of strokes with different intensity according to the needs of the subject.

A massage session may continue for 20-90 minutes depending on the type of massage and severity of pain. No matter what kind of massage you choose, you should feel relaxed and calm during and after the massage session.

Different **types of massage** include:

- *Swedish massage:* It uses long strokes, deep circular movements, kneading and tapping to energize you and to help you relax.
- *Deep massage:* This uses more forceful but slower strokes to target the deep layers of connective tissues and muscles of the hands. It helps with muscle damage from injuries.
- *Trigger point massage:* It is effective for areas of tight muscle fibers that occur after injury or overuse of those muscles.

- *Sports massage:* It is usually used for people involved in sports activities to help in treating injuries. It is similar to Swedish massage used for prevention of muscle injuries.

For arthritis patients of the hands and fingers, the most commonly used types of massage includes Deep Massage and Trigger point massage.

c) Hand self-massage: If the muscles around become tight, you can do self-massage by rubbing the area around your thumb with your other hand or by rolling your hand over the ball placed on any smooth surface.

d) The Benefits of Massage Therapy ease muscle spasms and muscle tension, decrease swelling and impaired joint mobility, and also improve blood circulation. It improves alertness levels and reduces stress and pain, it enhances sleep patterns and releases natural pain killers called endorphins from the body. Having soft muscles massaged by a trained therapist has many benefits including the release of knotted muscles and the improvement of blood circulation. Massage results in enhanced immune response with decreased stress hormones and increased "feel good" transmitters called serotonin. But despite the benefits of massage therapy, it is not a replacement for the regular medical opinion. Be sure to follow standard treatment plans and inform your doctor about the massage therapy.

e) Hypnosis*:* It is considered as a very important alternative therapy for pain management in Arthritis. It is very effective in reducing the intensity of pain in arthritic patients and to help the patients in reaching the deep state of relaxation. During hypnosis, qualified and experienced specialists help the subject to enter in a trance-like state of deep concentration. Hypnosis therapy deeply relaxes you and leaves your unconscious mind open for suggestions that might help in improving your health and to encourage changes in your behavior to relieve your symptoms of pain of arthritis in the hands and fingers. Hypnotherapy actually helps in pain reduction by changing the levels of the biochemical in the body that intensifies or causes the pain sensation. There is good evidence that the hypnosis technique is safe for arthritis pain and reduces the pain and anxiety associated with arthritis of the hands and fingers.

f) Herbal*:* This is the use of plants or plant extracts in the treatment of diseases. Conventional medicine uses only active ingredients of the plant but herbal therapy uses the whole plant in treatment with the belief that the mixture of all the chemicals in the whole plant will work in synergy to give a more prominent effect. Herbs used in the treatment of arthritis of the hands and fingers have different effects as some are good for *relaxing* the tense muscles of the hands, some for *improving sleep* quality by making you relax and calm, and some are effective at *soothing pain* associated with arthritis. Some have *anti-inflammatory properties* and others are used to *improve energy* and some have *painkilling* properties.

Some of the herbs that are efficient in treating arthritis of the hands and fingers include: Boswellis, Devil's claw, Rosehip, Capsaicin, and white willow bark.

- **Capsaicin:** Cayenne pepper contains capsaicin that has healing properties in many chronic diseases. It acts by depleting the nerves of a biochemical substance P, which transmits a pain message to the brain, thus resulting in reduced pain severity associated with arthritis. Commercially available topical creams containing Capsaicin are available as topical pain relievers. 0.025% Capsaicin creams are effective in pain management.

- **White Willow Bark:** Salicylate drugs were first derived from white willow bark, which is a milder, natural version of aspirin. Extract containing 60 to 100 mg of salicin per dose is effective in relieving mild arthritis pain of the hands and fingers.
- **Devil's Claw:** It is a medicinal plant native to Africa and contains iridoid glycosides that play a very effective role in reducing arthritis pain and improves results in mild to severe cases. Capsules with 400mg of *Harpagophytum* extract containing 1.5% iridoid glucosides content is sufficient in reducing pain severity.

The use of herbal medicines is safe but sometimes may cause sleeplessness, stomach upset, and pain in muscles and joints. When taken along with other medication they may interfere with medicines, so always consult your doctor and herbal practitioner to avoid any mishap.

g) Meditation*:*

Meditation is a simple and fast way to reduce stress and to relax you from the stress caused by pain. It calms you and restores your inner peace, resulting in enhanced physical and emotional well-being. It brings more relaxation and stress reduction in pain management of arthritis of the hands and fingers. It helps with pain perception by slowing the heart rate and breathing of the subject and concentrating on a sound called Mantra, resulting in decreased depression and anxiety caused by the pain associated with arthritis.

Ways to meditate include the following:

- *Guided Meditation:* In this type of meditation, the mental images of the places or situations are formed that you find relaxing. Other senses like smells, sounds, sights, and textures can also be used for this purpose.

- *Mindfulness Meditation:* This type of meditation involves increased acceptance and awareness of living in the present. The focus of this meditation is the experience during the flow of your breath; you observe different thoughts but ignore them without judging them.

- *Mantra Meditation:* In this type of meditation, distracting thoughts are prevented by silently repeating the calming words, phrases and thoughts.

- *Transcendental Meditation:* In this type of meditation, conscious awareness is narrowed by using your mantra, which could be any word, phrase or sound to eliminate all thoughts from the mind.

Studies have shown that people who regularly practiced Transcendental Meditation have milder stress responses. Few of the ways to practice mediation include deep breathing, engaging in a prayer, repeating a mantra, walking and meditating, scanning your body to become aware of different sensations, and listening to sacred music or reading poems.

h) Chiropractic: Chiropractic therapy in hand arthritis involves the passive joint manipulation. It involves passive joint movements of the fingers and thumb that are performed within the comfortable range of the subject. Chiropractic treatment helps in decreasing pain of the joints, helps in muscle spasms and improves the strength and functioning of joints.

i) Homeopathy: Homeopathy is based on the principle "like treats like" so for a swollen and tender joint remedy use bee stings which can cause swollen and tender swellings. Homeopathic medicines that are used for arthritis in the hands and fingers desensitize the immune system and control further joint damage. Homeopathic medicines reduce fatigue and inflammation in a very natural way and produce fewer side effects. The homeopathic system aims to clear out the disease from the body and not just suppress the disease or to give temporary relief. Duration of treatment may vary according to the severity of the disease, and the extent of damage.

Anemia occurred in Arthritis is treated very effectively with Ferrum Metallicum. Medicines that are used to treat Arthritis of the hands and fingers includes: Caulophyllum, Colchicum, Carcinocin, Rhus Tox etc.

j) Hydrotherapy*:* It is one of the Alternative therapies used for the treatment of Arthritis of the hands and fingers. It involves immersing part of the body or the whole body in water to reduce pain and to improve mobility. **Hydrotherapy** includes:

-Mineral baths

-Water-jet massage

-Bathing in heated water

-Cold Water therapy

-Whirlpool bath for Athletic injuries

-Ice for sprains

-Aquatic exercise

Hydrotherapy helps because water provides resistance, warmth, and support; it improves muscle strength and helps in pain reduction. Hydrotherapy is often combined with other conventional treatments for pain management. It improves the blood circulation and enhances the feeling of well being, without putting any stress on your painful joints.

Hydrotherapy for RA: Hydrotherapy is effective for RA patients to treat joint stiffness and pain associated with RA of the hands and fingers. The swelling in joints is decreased with hydrotherapy. Warm water is effective for improving mobility in affected joints by decreasing the swelling on the joints and soft tissues. In the water, gravitational forces of the body are reduced, giving a lighter load on the joints. Hydrotherapy with warm water also increases blood flow, which results in excessive oxygen rich blood to the body areas that need more oxygen. Warm water is muscle soothing and helps to release tension related to Arthritis.

Hydrotherapy for OA: It is effective for OA patients also as Water buoyancy allows easy joint movement by reducing the pressure on your joints. It is an excellent choice of treatment for people with painful joints and helps in range of motion exercise.

h) Alexander technique*:* It is the technique that eliminates the bad habits of posture, movements and muscle tension and improves the body position and movements.

i) Yoga*:* Yoga is a mind-body practice that includes relaxation, stretching exercises and controlled breathing. Someone affected by hand arthritis may not want to move the joint for the fear that the pain will increase but it is best to move that painful joint gently. Yoga has different styles, forms and intensities, out of which *Hatha Yoga* is the best choice with slow and easy movements for stress management associated with Arthritis pain in hands and wrists.

j) Mushtika Bandhana (Hand Clenching): This yoga asana is particularly useful in Arthritis of the hands and fingers. The Hand Clenching Asana provides the primary benefits of restoring or developing grip of the hands and also strengthens the joints of the hands and fingers. To perform this, sit comfortably on a chair with an erect back and put an arm out in front at shoulder level, parallel to the ground. With the thumb facing upwards, make a fist with all the fingers inserted into the thumb. Follow the movement along with breathing and when you inhale, open your fist to stretch all the fingers. When you exhale, again make a fist and repeat this process for 8-10 times on both hands.

Squeezing a stress ball is another way to improve the grip strength and to relieve pain and reduce inflammation in subjects with arthritis of hands.

If you are at risk of developing hand arthritis: In the stepwise approach to yoga, the cat/cow pose bearing weight on the hands, upward/downward facing dog pose and all arm balancing poses are helpful in maintaining good range of movement in the joints of your hands over time. A variety of hand seals, or hasta mudras can strengthen your fingers in a non-weight bearing way.

Those who have already developed hand arthritis: Less-weight bearing asana are important. Aids to permit inclusion of weight bearing asana includes specialized gloves with rubber cushions for the heel of the hands, as well as circular cushions, and rounded blocks called Yoga Jellies.

The benefits of Yoga therapy for hand arthritis include: Stress reduction, management of chronic conditions with severe pain, reduces blood pressure, and improves the heart function and overall fitness of the body.

k) Aromatherapy: Aromatherapy is a holistic approach to health and well being by using scents and aromas derived from the plant kingdom. It utilizes aromatic substances, mainly essential oils, in the treatment of arthritis. A qualified aroma-therapist selects the essential oils according to the patient's individual needs. You can inhale oils, or use them in the bath. Massaging into the skin with these oils helps in muscular pains, rheumatism, and poor circulation after diluting the oils in carrier oil. Lavender is used for the relief of muscle spasms.

The following formula is good for arthritis:

Essential oil of Lavender: 3 drops

Essential oil of Rosewood: 3 drops,

Essential oil Roman Camomile: 2 drops

dissolved in carrier oil of 20 ml of Sweet Almond.

This formulation is kept in a dark amber glass bottle and stored in a cool dry place. Gently massage the affected area of the hands to have relief from pain.

Combination for RA: Treatment includes the following blend of essential oils:

German chamomile: 5 drops

Rosemary Chemotype verbenone: 3 drops

Yellow birch: 4 drops

Geranium: 4 drops in 30 ml of Carrier oil of Rosehip with 5 ml of infused Saint John's Wort added in it. This formula has soothing analgesic and anti-inflammatory effects on painful swollen joints.

Aromatherapy is effective and safe for pain management in arthritis of hands and fingers as aromatherapy massage gives relief for several days, if not weeks. However, it is harmful in large quantities and may cause occasional allergic reactions.

l) Osteopathy*:* It involves gentle manual stretching, traction and mobility techniques on joints, muscles and ligaments. Exercises to do at home, and in warm water or salt baths may also be recommended to reduce swelling and pain and to improve the range of movements and mobility of joints of the hands and fingers.

The aims of Osteopathy are to provide immediate relief from symptoms, improve mobility, reduce pain and swelling, assist in rehabilitation and to educate people on how to improve the quality of life through diet, exercise and posture.

m) Music Therapy*:* Music is like exercise and what you listen to does not matter as long as you are really involved. Music can decrease the pain, disability, and depression that occur in arthritic patients. Music is a powerful and magical medium as it can inspire all our senses. It has the power to soothe and comfort us. Music therapy also has influence on pain perception, blood pressure, and respiratory rates and also on the immune system.

There is a direct link between specific sounds and different parts of the body. Recent studies show that with slow-tempo classical music, pain may ease and faster compositions stimulate the heart rate and nervous system. While listening to this type of music, you will have more painful feelings. Pay attention to your heart rate and breathing while listening to the music, feel relaxed with the music and let the stress melt away.

Music stimulates those areas of the brain that cause the release of the body's own painkillers. Music stimulates the periaqueductal gray area in the brain, in which we have our own pain relieving mechanism. Imaging studies have shown that music stimulates the pleasure center of the brain, and increases dopamine and substance P levels of brain, resulting in the feeling of enjoyment and pain inhibition. Brain scan evidences also show that music blocks the amygdala part of the brain that is responsible for negative emotions including stress.

n) Magnet therapy*:* Magnets produce a certain type of energy known as a Magnetic field. There are two types of magnets: electromagnet and static. A static magnet has health benefits and produces an unchanging magnetic field. Electromagnets produce a changing field when a current is passed through it.

The theory about how magnets work includes the idea that static magnets may change cell function and increase the oxygen and blood supply to the tissues. Static magnets are placed under the clothing or placed on the skin.

Magnet therapy comes in the form of a necklace, bracelets, inserts or disks and is helpful in treating Arthritic pain.

Chapter 9) Understanding the Importance of Self-Assessment

Understanding the importance of Self-Assessment in Arthritics of he Hands & Fingers

"*The greatest revolution of our time is the knowledge that human beings, by changing the inner attitudes of their minds, can transform the outer aspects of their lives*". – William James

Self-assessment starts with acknowledging your potential risk factors. Your age, gender, medical history, family history, obesity, ethnic origin and exposure of your hands and fingers to harmful factors are significant in estimating your chances. People need to be educated about the importance of self-awareness in arthritis. The following steps can make a lot of difference in reducing the agony of the patients on one hand and on the other hand it can save millions of dollars spent each year on treating arthritis.

-Support organizations in communicating the benefits of self-awareness to patients.

-Assist health professionals with determining the cost patients can save through self-awareness.

-Promote peer learning among nurses, doctors and allied healthcare providers.

-Emphasis on promoting arthritis self-awareness to low-income groups of the community, as they are the ones most likely to benefit from it.

-Arrange small workshops, as they tend to have higher completion and compliance rates compared to anything else. For greater success, local philanthropic organizations, colleges, universities and community-based organizations can be engaged to deliver this important message about self-awareness in arthritis.

This will not only yield good results for arthritis prevention, but the same can be done for other chronic illnesses as well. This will encourage patients to take some of the easiest steps to the prevention of hand and wrist arthritis.

Special attention should be given to the hands and fingers; try to keep them warm and safe all the time. Wear gloves (light cotton knit), even if the temperature is slightly lower than normal. Hot paraffin treatment is a very good way to keep arthritic hands and fingers warm. Always try to use stemware instead of normal drinking glasses. Large stem glasses are always easier to grip. Make it part of your routine to exercise daily under a professional therapist's instructions. Joint and muscle movements are significant for prevalence purposes.

1) Is there a Cure for Arthritis in the Hands & Fingers?

Those who suffer from arthritis usually present this question to their physician. Unfortunately, there is no definitive treatment of arthritis as it has multiple causes and some of its causes are still being studied. Healthcare providers are treating symptoms of wrist or hand arthritis to the best of their abilities. We can say that medicines tend to control arthritis rather than cure it.

Hand therapy is the most suggested and safest treatment for hand or wrist arthritis. Hand therapy is very helpful in maintaining mobility and reducing pain. For fingers, there are many surgeries available that are currently in use but people should opt for food supplements to start with. Also, there are many complications and side effects related to surgeries. Food supplements have been showing positive results in reducing stiffness and pain in most of the patients. A good thing about these supplements is that they are available easily and can be purchased without a doctor's prescription (over-the-counter drug). Patients with chronic illness can use technology to their benefit. Use an ergonomically designed keyboard and mouse, wear designed gloves for arthritic patients and specially manufactured grip providing daily utensils for firm grip and comfortable eating and drinking.

2) Myths Regarding Arthritis

Many people out there are unaware of the fact that there are hundreds of different types of arthritis. Arthritis is not only pain and stiffness, but it is a musculoskeletal disorder. It can also seriously harm other internal organs of our body. Getting diagnosed early is the right approach to start treatment. Physicians and researchers are continuously working for successful and effective treatments. The United States is spending more than $130 million annually on the treatment and prevalence sector.

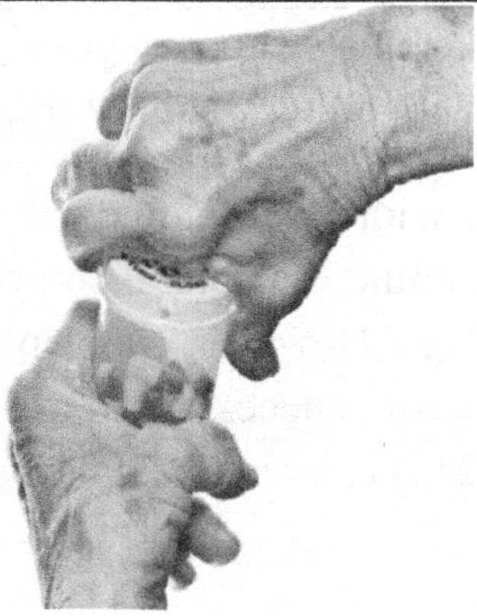

Myth # 1: A very common term "there is no cure" is used for arthritis, particularly for those with hands and fingers' arthritis. We can't do anything about it either. However, it's not true. We can do a lot of stuff to reduce the symptoms. Begin with weight loss to minimize the pressure on the joints, either hand or foot joints. Daily exercise, a planned diet and proper medications are ideal to successfully curing your illness.

Myth # 2- Diet has nothing to do with arthritis treatment of hands and fingers. Fish, meat, olive oil, vegetables and all food items; these are rich in omega-3 fatty acids. "Keeping your overall health in better position is very important to counter arthritis symptoms" says *Lona Sandon, RD and spokeswoman for the Academy of Nutrition and Dietetics.* So next time you eat, don't forget to add all such food items with anti-inflammation qualities. Also remember to intake the daily-prescribed amount of calcium as well.

Myth # 3- We can't exercise while having symptoms in the hands and fingers. This is totally not true. In fact, not exercising can increase the pain with time. Small and limited joint and muscle movements are very important to stabilize mobility in fingers. Limited motion and low impact-ranged exercises are instructed to patients by therapists. Yoga is getting much more popular amoung patients with all types of arthritis.

Myth # 4- Supplements with glucosamine will naturally recover my joints. Glucosamine is a natural compound that is present in joints and cartilage. However, supplements are not enough for treatment; rather it is necessary to inject it in the knee for any potential benefit. This can only be done by a professional and not at home.

Myth # 5- Cracking knuckles and joints can cause arthritis later on in life. The good news is that this is not true. There is no clinical evidence of any such incident. Nevertheless, cracking knuckles can be annoying. It may result in normal pain and stiffness of joints. Avoid making a habit of such movements that may damage your joints in any possible manner.

3) Duration for Successful Treatments

Accurate treatment tailored specifically to each patient depending upon the severity of their illness is the key to successful recovery and reduction of inflammation in joints of arthritic hands and arthritic fingers. Treatment may involve many steps and several procedures like non-drug massage therapies, medications and surgeries. We can estimate the duration of recovery if the target of treatment is the reduction of signs and symptoms and an increase in mobility and the patient's overall quality of life. The initial target of every treatment is to stop inflammation to avoid further complications. Successful treatment may take from 3 to 6 months, depending upon the condition of patient.

According to a research study conducted in August 2011*(Published in final edited form as: J Rheumatol. 2011*

August; 38(8): 1680–1688. Published online 2011 May 15. doi: 10.3899/jrheum.101196, PMCID: PMC3149716, NIHMSID: NIHMS288635) patients with arthritis in the hands and fingers can be at risk of joint fracture. Joint fractures in such patients can occur due to any accidental force exerted on their hand or fingers. This study concluded that special importance should be given to patients for fracture prevention.

A rehabilitation program must include a professional therapist who will assess your condition and assist your mobility and flexibility in both hands and fingers. All rehabilitation methods can be tough in the beginning, causing you discomfort. However, with time you will be able to counter inflammation in your joints. Most patients recover quickly and return to their normal lives with an easily available, wide range of helping gadgets.

Chapter 10) Professionals at High Risk

Professionals at High Risk of Arthritis in Hands & Fingers

1) High Risk Professionals

Jobs that require you to make repetitive movements of the hands, fingers and thumbs on a daily basis for a long period of time, year after year, put you at an increased risk of arthritis in the hands and fingers. It implies that arthritis of the hands and fingers can strike professionals in fields from manufacturing to music if they don't take the necessary precautionary measures seriously.

Mostly people working in professions involving heavy physical labor with repetitive movements such as: stooping, pulling, pushing, lifting, carrying, twisting, or reaching will be at very high risk of developing arthritis in their hands and fingers. Farming and construction are two very common high-risk occupations in the USA, there are others (heavy industry and occupations with repetitive hand movements that stress and eventually damage joints)

Apart from construction and textile workers, which are well-documented risk professions, some less known and unexpected professions, such as particular musicians (Pianists, guitarists or flute musicians) and office workers like typists are also high-risk professions for arthritis in the hands. Some of the most common risk professions are listed below with a brief description of movements resulting in the development of hand or finger arthritis.

a) Construction: Working in the construction industry poses many arthritic risks. Incorrect lifting of weights and machinery without the right equipment is the most common arthritis risk factor for construction industry workers. Another cause of arthritis is using tools that vibrate. People who use air hammers routinely have a higher instance of getting problems in their hands, wrists, and fingers. The major problems are arthritis and muscle injuries. The only way to reduce your chances of developing hand arthritis is to perform different tasks so that you can avoid doing the same repetitive movements for better arthritis prevention. Consider taking frequent breaks if you are bound to perform a job that involves repetitive hand or finger movements.

b) Musicians: The life of a musician might be very appealing to those who like them and listen to their master pieces, but a melody or a symphony you admire is a product of sheer hard work that requires a lot of repetitive motion, which can lead to arthritis. Usually their joints, after years of practice, become flexible to allow certain movements but at the same time they are at an increased risk of injuring those joints. Arthritis prevention may vary from instrument to instrument. For example, a pianist needs to use a combination of wrist and finger exercises while a guitarist must learn to hold a guitar correctly to reduce strain on the wrist, elbow, and shoulder.

c) Typists/Writers: People doing excessive typing have an increased prevalence of finger and wrist arthritis. Although a writer has the luxury of using multiple ways of delivering his thoughts into print form as he may choose to hand write or record his stuff, still some writers suffer from wrist and finger arthritis due to the use of type writers and computer key boards excessively during writing. Office secretaries and typists don't have any such luxuries. They are expected to be fast and sharp in their work, which leads to injuries to their wrist joints and small joints in their fingers. Some common strategies to reduce the incidence of injuries include learning how to place your hands on the type writer or keyboard correctly, encouraging yourself to stay fit and healthy (which helps reduce strain on joints), and using wrist pads in work assignments to avoid aggravating an existing joint injury and arthritis symptoms. "The industry is not very well aware of the issues and needs to cut down on risks wherever possible.

d) Professional Athletes: Young adults pursuing their dreams in athletics and gymnastics put their joints under extreme stress and frequently end up with aching joints, but arthritis of the hands and fingers are as much a part of the deal in their later years. A weight lifter or a gymnast can end up with injuries to small and medium sized joints of the fingers, wrists and hand. Arthritis prevention must be customized according to the needs of specific sports. For example, professional hockey/ice hockey players must learn to fall in such a way as to avoid direct injuries to their wrists.

e) Dancers: Despite all its aesthetic beauties and refinements, over the years, dance can be one of the causes of arthritis in almost every joint. Ankles and hips are likely candidates for arthritis but certain types of dances, which involve exaggerated hand and finger movements may also induce arthritis symptoms in aged dancers.

f) Textile Workers: Textile workers working in mass production scenarios are bound to perform certain routine movements when operating machinery or packaging. For example, certain production line routines need workers to reach over their head. Following those routines is likely to produce arthritis from the shoulder to the hand. Good posture, minimizing stress on the hand and taking appropriate breaks can help ease the stress on joints and can reduce the chances of arthritis development.

g) Truck & Long Distance Drivers: These drivers are in a profession that is highly demanding on their bodies and limits physical activity as they spend most of their time sitting in their driving seats. In addition to limiting postural movements, their hands must remain alert all the time. This puts an enormous pressure on their wrists, fingers and hands. When we consider the repetition of the movement then they are on the worst side. Imagine you are driving for a week with only breaks for meals and rest or sleep. How much stress can your body take and for how long? It's just a matter of time until your joints give in to this stress.

Chapter 11) Arthritis – Give Yourself A Break

1) Risks of not resting our hands & fingers enough.

While exploring different methods of treatment for arthritic hands and fingers, we must understand the importance of resting our hands and fingers enough during work routines. Many patients take high doses of painkillers and antidepressants to reduce their pain and to counter their stress and depression. However, most of the arthritis patients fail to realize that they are not resting their hands and fingers enough while working. Affected arthritis individuals tend to get so busy on their computer that they forget to rest their hands and fingers for a long enough amount of time. We must understand that failing to do so can increase the severity and pain of existing arthritis symptoms. Patients in the initial stages of their illness can push themselves to permanent and more painful hand and finger injuries. Consequences to such ignorance can lead to permanent disability as well. The same theory is applicable to patients suffering from arthritis in their back, neck, shoulders, arms, wrist, legs and toes.

Nowadays, social media sites are so engaging that individuals can easily spend hours on the net chatting within their community without taking any break. Sometimes people skip their meal times during net surfing and chatting. There are abundant theories on the long-term side effects of too much use of electronic and gaming devices. Excessive use of such devices including computers can also be harmful to your eyesight and memory. Acute to severe headaches are a normal symptom for prolonged exposure to such devices.

Each individual suffering from similar illnesses has to schedule their use of computers and gaming devices. A planned routine is a good option but for frequent users this can be particularly hard as they can find it very difficult to take breaks between their gaming and computing sessions. For such users, using particular software that can remind them or even force them to take a break in between can be a perfect option and a healthier solution to their resting needs.

2) Office dangers for Arthritis patients

In office jobs, executives have to use computers on a daily basis for 3-5 hours and sometimes even more. This exaggerated use is even more alarming for patients of arthritis in hands, wrists and fingers working in these jobs. Daily usage can easily accelerate painful symptoms and the sufferings can be permanent rather than moving towards improvement. For professionals, painkillers, herb supplements, anti-inflammatory drugs and muscle relaxants are not a good option as such drugs can induce addiction in the patient. Patients find it impossible to recover from their deteriorating symptoms and rely solely on the painkillers for any significant relief in pain.

The severity of arthritic symptoms in hands, wrists, fingers and thumbs can permanently disable professionals and limit them from performing their duties. The consequences can even get worse with time if left unattended or untreated.

3) A Reliable Solution

There is no need for you to make the similar mistake of ignoring your resting needs between working. A simple and most suitable solution for professionals as well as home users of computers is the installation of a well renowned and result oriented application named "*Break Reminder Software*". The use of this software is so easy. Just install and run, as simple as that. It will help you recover your health and protect your joints and bones from further disintegration, providing you with enough breaks during your working hours without you even noticing its use.

4) Break Reminder Software:

www.breakremindersoftware.com *Break Reminder Software* will force you to take breaks while using your computer for long durations. Just double click the setup and it will be installed on your pc within seconds in 3 simple steps, just like any other window software.

How it Works: It is auto-run software that will start with the window. The software's basic functioning is manual regarding the setting up of breaks. This way you can setup breaks according to your needs. There is a tab named "Breaks". You can use this tab to select the duration of your break.

Note: You can disable this software anytime you want so its use is customizable. This application is user friendly just like a friend to help you get enough breaks and save you from stress and potential injuries.

Users' Review: A professional named Leah Hutchinson developed a repetitive strain injury in her neck, shoulders, arms, wrists and fingers. This strain happened due to nonstop use of a mouse and keyboard, typing for hours and working in the office. The pain in her whole body, especially in the hands and fingers was intolerable. "I had to visit my physician a number of times without having any improvement in my situation. I exercised daily and used all prescribed drugs but I was still in tears without any hope of escape from my strain. I began to wonder whether there was any cure for me or not. Then one day I came across this amazing and so easy to use application called *Break Reminder Software*. I now thank myself for installing this application as a solution to my pain. And now I am fully recovered from my illness and working like my old days. By creating mandatory breaks during typing and mouse use has helped me reduce my pain to zero" says Hutchinson.

Similar reviews can be heard for this software from thousands of satisfied users. Don Cowan a research IT-analyst and Kurt Edwards a game designer have both used this software and are very happy with the results. Remember! It is very critical for any arthritis and repetitive strain patient to prevent his/her body from extra burden and to rest enough during working. So get yourself a copy of *Break Reminder Software* and start using it today. This application is the right solution for all your resting needs.

Chapter 12) Helping the Patients

The best help that can be extended to an arthritis patient is to educate them about their disease, as this is the first step towards improving their quality of life. There are numerous assistive devices on the market to increase mobility, reduce physical limitations and reduce pain for patients with Arthritic hands and fingers. You or your loved one might reach a point of total disability. In this scenario, you must know all about different helping aids that can assist you in overcoming your work restrictions.

1) Self Care Tips

Self-care tip#1- Read more and more about Arthritic hands and fingers to understand your condition and the right tools to counter it successfully. There are a lot of online resources, e-books and medical data available to assist you.

Self-care tip#2- *Consult* your rheumatologist for all possible treatment options, he/she will guide you better after complete and proper diagnosis of your arthritis in hands and fingers. Your doctor is the right person to guide you to the best approach.

Self-care tip#3-Burden of chronic pain can be lethal; it can easily take away all the pleasures and hopes of your life. It is very important for you to stay motivated during the course of treatment. Brain and heart combination can be your secret to successfully counter your arthritis. Keep your focus on solutions rather than problems. Discuss your situation with friends and family as well in order to receive healthy and motivating responses.

Self-care tip#4- Pain in arthritic hands and arthritic fingers is inevitable. However, don't get bogged down and participate in your daily life activities that you enjoy most. You can opt for traveling, working, shopping, or engaging yourself in social and welfare activities.

Self-care tip#5- Medication is always a major tool of treatment for most patients with *Arthritis in hands and fingers*. There are many classes of drugs that are used in different scenarios for treating arthritis. These medications include; Cox-2 selective inhibitors, NSAIDs, DMARDs, analgesics, response modifiers, ointments and creams. Utilize prescribed combinations timely to gain their right effects.

2) Frequently Faced Problems & their Simple Solutions

The following table explains some of the most common problems encountered in everyday life with simple and practical solutions.

Activity	Problem	Solution
Writing	Weak grip because of painful wrist & fingers.	Use a pen with a chunky rubber grip and keep a light, relaxing grip during the writing.
Peeling	Gripping and turning the peeler.	Choose a wide handled peeler
Washing/drying back, neck & feet	Reach is limited due to pain.	Wash with a long handled sponge and use lightweight dry towel.
Turning a key	Gripping & turning at 90 degrees or more.	Fit a handle to your key for better grip.
Picking things up from the floor	Reaching down	Use a pick up tool

3) Searching for More Ways

a) How it works- Communicate and meditate properly. All those physical activities that were once taken for granted are now difficult to perform. Adapt relaxing techniques to reduce related pain and stress. Stress can have a negative impact on your personality. It will only increase your misery, nothing else.

b) Online equipment shopping- The first rule of coping with pain in hands and fingers is to keep them safe from strain. A specialist in the field will guide you on how to do several general tasks differently, in order to minimize your effort and use of hands and fingers. You can follow professional advice and related tools to perform many tasks easily. There is a wide range of assistive products that can be used to reduce pain and increase mobility.

-Special mugs and cups

-Clothing and bib protectors

-Bathing gloves

-Flexible cup holder

-Gas Bud-E Hands Free Fueling Clip

-Arthritis Gloves

-Soap Holder Long Handle Bath Sponge

-Arthritis finger splint-First-aid devices

-Utensil hand clip

-Over-bed tables for easy approach

-No slip strips

-Perfect grip utensil strap

-Straw holder

-Universal hand clip

-Non-slippery silicon mats

-Handy bar

-Headrest Grab Handles

4) Links to websites

We have already mentioned in this book that there are many helpful websites thar offer important resources about arthritis (hand and finger), along with options of online shopping of helping tools for hand and fingers. Listed below are a few of the most visited websites for online information and buying products.

http://www.arthritis.org/

http://www.howto.co.uk/wellbeing/rheumatoid-treatment/equipment_and_adaptations/

http://www.arthritissupplies.com

http://www.rashop.co.uk/

http://www.afstore.org/site/index-afstore.html

http://www.aidsfordailyliving.com.au/learning/cat/arthritis

http://www.aidsfordailyliving.com.au/learning/cat/arthritis/

http://www.alibaba.com/showroom/arthritis-equipment.html

http://www.homemedi.com/dgrheumatoid-arthritis.htm

http://www.healthtalkonline.org/disability/Rheumatoid_Arthritis/Topic/2236/

http://rawarrior.com/tag/shopping-with-rheumatoid-arthritis/

http://www.arthritistoday.org/what-you-can-do/staying-active/gadgets-and-gear/golf-accessories.php

http://www.arthritistoday.org/what-you-can-do/everyday-solutions/do-it-easier/driving-and-travel/arthritis-friendly-car-shopping.php

http://www.niagaratherapy.co.uk/

http://www.storesonline.com/site/371928/page/45029/rheumatoid

http://www.giveasyoulive.com/search/stores

http://www.chemistwarehouse.com.au/healthinfo/article.asp?ID=1482

http://www.health.harvard.edu/special_health_reports/Arthritis

http://www.allegromedical.com/blog/living-young-despite-rheumatoid-arthritis-patricias-story-2866.html

http://www.dailymail.co.uk/health/article-2177031/Arthritis-remedies-Experts-reveal-treatments-really-work.html

http://www.amazon.co.uk/Living-Rheumatoid-Arthritis-Hopkins-Health/dp/0801871476

http://www.tractorsupply.com/know-how_Lifestyle_protect-yourself-fom-osteoarthritis

http://www.webmd.com/rheumatoid-arthritis/guide/assistive-devices

http://www.ncpad.org/112/869/Rheumatoid~Arthritis~and~Exercise

http://www.arthritissolutions.com.au/

http://usmedicbay.com/catalog/Weight_Loss/Xenical.htm

http://marlenadelacroix.com/rheumatoid-arthritis-medication/

http://www.walgreens.com/pharmacy/specialtypharmacy.jsp

http://www.physioneeds.biz/ProductDetail.aspx/Actimove_Wrist_Brace_/SUP120

http://www.rafapal.com/?p=36362

http://health.nytimes.com/health/guides/disease/rheumatoid-arthritis/diagnosis.html

http://health.howstuffworks.com/wellness/aging/retirement/10-exercises-for-people-with-arthritis.htm

https://www.ncmedical.com/

http://www.sportsmedicineclinicdelhi.com/link.htm

Suggested Studies

3 Minutes to a Pain-Free Life: The Groundbreaking Program for Total Body ...by Joseph Weisberg, Heidi Shink

Concordance Repertory of the Materia Medica by William D. Gentry, William Daniel Gentry

Splinting the Hand and Upper Extremity: Principles and Processedited by MaryLynn A. Jacobs, Noelle Austin, Noelle M. Austin

Diagnostic Imaging of the Hand by Rainer Schmitt, Ulrich Lanz

Arthritis - by John D. Clough

Healthy Living Series- Arthritis

Conquering Arthritis by Barbara D. Allan

Arthritis: 300 Tips for Making Life Easier by Shelley Peterman Schwarz

The First Year--rheumatoid Arthritis: An Essential Guide for the Newly Diagnosed by M. E. A. McNeil

Arthritis Research: Treatment and Management edited by Frank H. Columbus

Rheumatoid Arthritisedited by E. William St. Clair, David S. Pisetsky, Barton F. Haynes

Rheumatoid Arthritis by Marc C. Hochberg, Alan J. Silman, Josef S. Smolen, Michael E. Weinblatt, Michael H. Weisman

How to Treat Arthritis with Sex and Alcohol: And Other Breakthroughs and ... by Carter V. Multz, MD F. A. C. P. F. A. C. R. Carter V Multz

Arthritis: questions you have ... answers you need.

Further Studies

*SSH Manual of Hand Surgery by Warren C. Hammert, Martin I. Boyer, David J. Bozentka, Ryan Patrick Calfee

Wolters Kluwer Health | Lippincott Williams & Wilkins

---

*Easing the Pain of Arthritis Naturally: Everything You Need to Know to

By Earl L. Mindell, Ph.D., Mindell R.PH. Ph.D., Earl L.

Read How You Want
YOUR CUSTOMIZED BOOK SOURCE

---

*Arthritis: 300 Tips for Making Life Easier

By Shelley Peterman Schwarz

Read How You Want
YOUR CUSTOMIZED BOOK SOURCE

---

*Rheumatoid Arthritis and Proteus

By Alan Ebringer

Springer

---

*Arthritis-

DK Publishing, 20-Jul-2009 - Health & Fitness

Helping readers live with arthritis and its long term complications, this guide covers everything from medical definitions of the various forms of arthritis to all aspects of treating the condition. Discusses pros and cons of treatment options available. Covers diet, exercise, medication, surgery, and many more.

Publisher	DK Publishing, 2009
ISBN	0756667542, 9780756667542
Length	224 pages

*Arthritis:

Improve Your Health, Ease Pain, and Live Life to the Full

Expert advice based on up-to-the-minute research, from specialists in arthritis careEverything you need to know about arthritis to improve your health, ease pain, and live life to the full is covered in this updated new edition. Learn about every type of arthritis, from juvenile to rheumatoid and osteoarthritis arthritis.

Dorling Kindersley, 03-Aug-2009 - Arthritis - 224 pages

*Atlas of Psoriatic Arthritis

edited by P. J. Mease, Philip Helliwell

Springer

Springer. Copyright.

*Arthritis in Black and White

By Anne C. Brower, Donald J. Flemming

---

*The Great Physician's Rx for Arthritis

By Jordan Rubin

THOMAS NELSON
Since 1798

Imaging of Arthritis and Metabolic Bone Disease: Expert Consult - Online

By Barbara N. W. Weissman

---

*Diagnostic Imaging of the Hand

By Rainer Schmitt, Ulrich Lanz

Thieme

---

*Top 3 Differentials in Radiology: A Case Review

By William O'Brien

Thieme

---

*Psoriatic Arthritis

By Dafna D. Gladman, Vinod Chandran

Oxford University Press. Copyright.

*What to Do when the Doctor Says It's Rheumatoid Arthritis: Cure Your Pain ...

By Harry D. Fischer, Winnie Yu

Fair Winds. Copyright.

*Rehabilitation of the Hand and Upper Extremity, 2-Volume Set: Expert Consult

By Terri M. Skirven, A. Lee Osterman, Jane Fedorczyk, Peter C. Amadio

Elsevier Health Sciences. Copyright.

*Arthritis in Color: Advanced Imaging of Arthritis

By Michael A. Bruno, Gary E. Gold, Timothy J. Mosher

Elsevier Health Sciences. Copyright.

*High-Resolution Radiographs of the Hand

By Giuseppe Guglielmi, Wilfred C. G. Peh, Mario Cammisa

Springer. Copyright.

*Differential Diagnosis in Conventional Radiology

By Francis Burgener, Martti Kormano

Thieme

Thieme. Copyright.

---

*Rheumatoid Arthritis: Early Diagnosis and Treatment

By John J. Cush, Michael E. Weinblatt, Arthur Kavanaugh

Professional Communications. Copyright.

---

*Juvenile Arthritis: The Ultimate Teen Guide

By Kelly Rouba

Scarecrow Press, Inc.

Scarecrow Press. Copyright.

---

*The Cleveland Clinic Guide to Arthritis

By John Clough

KAPLAN

Kaplan Publishing. Copyright.

---

*Rheumatoid Arthritis: New Insights for the Healthcare Professional:

2011 Edition

ScholarlyEditions. Copyright.

---

*3 Minutes to a Pain-Free Life: The Groundbreaking Program for Total Body pain prevention and rapid relief

By Joseph Weisberg, Heidi Shink

SIMON & SCHUSTER
SIMONANDSCHUSTER.COM

---

*Post Mortem: Solving History's Great Medical Mysteries

By Philip A. Mackowiak

ACP PRESS

---

*The Arthritis Help-book:

A Tested Self-Management Program for Coping with Arthritis and Fibromyalgia

The world's leading guide to arthritis and fibromyalgia-including up-to-date information on all available treatments, medications, and surgeries. Proven techniques to reduce pain and increase dexterity. How to build a calcium-rich diet? and maintain a healthy weight. Designing an exercise program to match specific needs.

Kate Lorig, James F. Fries

A great hand book for sufferers of arthritis. I would recommend it for those who suffer from this disease or their loved ones. Helpful hints regarding medication, exercise and diet.

---

*Skeletal Radiology: The Bare Bones

By Felix S. Chew

Wolters Kluwer Health | Lippincott Williams & Wilkins

---

*Exercise and Chronic Disease: An Evidence-based Approach

---

edited by John Saxton (Prof.)

Taylor & Francis. Copyright.

---

*A Complete Illustrated Guide to Cooking with Arthritis: Helping the physical challenged regain their independence in the kitchen

By Melinda Winner

Tate Publishing. Copyright.

---

*Arthritis For Dummies

By Barry Fox, Nadine Taylor, Jinoos Yazdany, Dr Sarah Brewer

WILEY
Publishers Since 1807

John Wiley & Sons.

References

* Lawrence RC, Helmick CG, Arnett FC et al. Estimates of the prevalence of arthritis and selected musculoskeletal disorders in the United States. Arthritis Rheum 1998; 41:778– 99.

* Yelin E and Callahan LF. The economic cost and social and psychological impact of musculoskeletal conditions. Arthritis Rheum 1995; 38:1351– 1362.

* Fries JF, Spitz P, Kraines RG et al. Measurement of patient outcome in arthritis. Arthritis Rheum 1980; 23:137– 145.

* Lequesne MG, Mery C, Samson M et al. Indexes of severity for osteoarthritis of the hip and knee. Scand J Rheumatol 1987; 65S:85– 89.

* Bellamy N, Buchanan WW, Goldsmith H et al. Validation study of WOMAC: A health status instrument for measuring clinically important patient relevant outcomes to antirheumatic drug therapy in patients with osteoarthritis of the hip or knee. J Rheumatol 19; 15:1833– 1840.

* Wyke B. The neurology of joints: a review of general prinicples. Clin Rheum Dis 1981; 7:223– 239.

* Schaible HG and Grubb BD. Afferent and spinal mechanisms of joint pain. Pain 1993; 55:5– 54.

* Melzack R, Wall PD: Pain mechanisms: A new theory. Science. 150:971– 979, 1965.

6. Dexter D, Brandt K. Distribution and predictors of depressive symptoms in osteoarthritis. J Rheumatol 1993; 21:279– 286.

7. Davis MA, Ettinger WH, Neuhaus JM, Barclay JD, Segal MR. Correlates of knee pain among U.S. adults with and without radiographic knee osteoarthritis. J Rheumatol 1992; 19(12): 1943– 1948.

* Wegener ST. Psychosocial aspects of rheumatic disease: The developing biopsychosocial framework. Curr Opin Rheumatol 1991; 3:300– 304.

* Summers MN, Haley WE, Reveille JD, Alarcon GS. Radiographic assessment and psychologic variables as predictors of pain and functional impairment in osteoarthritis of the knee or hip. Arthritis Rheum 1988; 31:204– 209.

* Lorig K, Chastain, RL, Ung E, et al. Development and evaluation of a scale to measure perceived self-efficacy in people with arthritis. Arthritis Rheum 1989; 32:37– 44.

* Crook J, Rideout E , Browne G. The prevalence of pain complaints in a general population. Pain 1984; 18:299– 314.

* McCarthy C, Cushnaghan J, Dieppe P. Osteoarthritis. In: Wall PD, Melzack R (eds.), Textbook of Pain, 3rd edition. Edinburgh: Churchill Livingstone, 1994.

* Fort J. Celecoxib, a COX– 2– specific inhibitor: The clinical data. Am J Orthopedics 1999; 28(3Supp):13– 18.

* Harden RN, Bruehl SP, Backonja MM. The use of opioids in treatment of chronic pain: An examination of the ongoing controversy. J Back Musculoskel Rehab 1997; 9:155– 180.

* Ytterberg SR, Maren ML, Woods SR. Codeine and oxycodone use in patients with chronic rheumatic disease pain. Arthritis Rheum 1998; 41(9):1603– 1612

* Arnoldi CC, Djurhuus JC, Heerfordt J et al. Intraosseous phlebography, intraosseous pressure measurements and 99mTc polyphosphate scintigraphy in patients with various painful conditions in the hip and knee. Acta Orthopaedica Scandinavica 1980; 51:19– 28.

* Brandt KD and Slemenda CW. In: Schumacher HR, Klippel JH, Koopman WJ (eds.), Primer on the Rheumatic Diseases, 10th edition. Atlanta: The Arthritis Foundation, 1993.

* American College of Rheumatology Ad Hoc Committee on Clinical Guidelines. Guidelines for the initial evaluation of the adult patient with acute musculoskeletal symptoms. Arthritis Rheum 1996; 39:1– 8

* Williams HJ, Ward JR, Egger MJ et al. Comparison of naproxen and acetaminophen in a two-year study of treatment of osteoarthitis of the knee. Arthritis Rheum 1993; 36:1196– 1206.

* Bradley JD, Brandt KD, Katz BP et al. Comparison of an antiinflammatory dose of ibuprofen, an analgesic dose of ibuprofen, and acetaminophen in the treatment of patients with osteoarthritis of the knee. N Eng J Med 1991; 325:87– 91.

* McCormack K. Nonsteroidal antiinflammatory drugs and spinal nociceptive processing. Pain 1994; 59:9– 43.

* Hochberg MC, Altman RD, Brandt KD et al. Guidelines for the medical management of osteoarthritis. Arthritis Rheum 1995; 38:1535– 1546.

* Mao J, Price DD, Mayer DJ. Experimental mononeuropathy reduces the antinociceptive effects of morphine: Implications for common intracellular mechanisms involved in morphine tolerance and neuropathic pain. Pain 1995; 61:353– 364.

* Katz WA. The role of tramadol in the management of musculoskeletal pain. Today's Therapeutic Trends 1995; 13:177–186.

* Scnitzer TJ, Kamin M, Olson WH. Tramadol allows reduction of naproxen dose among patients with naproxen-responsive osteoarthritis pain. A randomized, double-blind, placebo controlled study. Arthritis Rheum 1999:42(7):1370– 1377.

* Wollheim FA. Current pharmacologic treatment of osteoarthritis. 1996; 52Suppl3:27– 38.

* Algozzine et al. Trolamine salicylate cream in osteoarthritis of the knee. JAMA 1982; 247:1311– 1313.

* Acupuncture. NIH Consensus Statement. 1997 Nov 3– 4; 15(5):1–

* McAlindon TE, Felson DT, Zhang Y et al. Relation of dietary intake and serum levels of vitamin D to progression of osteoarthritis of the knee among participants of the Framingham study. Ann Int Med 1996; 125:353– 359.

* Monks R. Psychotropic drugs. In:Wall PD, Melzack R (eds.), Textbook of Pain, 3rd edition. Edinburgh: Churchill Livingtone, 1994.

* Carette S, McCain GA, Bell DA, Fam AG. Evaluation of amitriptyline in primary fibrositis : A double-blind, placebo-controlled study. Arthritis Rheum 1986; 29:655– 659.

* Deal CL, Schnitzer TJ, Lipstein E et al. Treatment of arthritis with topical capsaicin: A double-blind trial. Clin Ther 1991; 13:383– 395.

* Monga, Trilok (Editor); Grabois, Martin (Editor). Pain Management in Rehabilitation.

New York, NY, USA: Demos Medical Publishing, 2002. p 232.

http://site.ebrary.com/lib/westthames/Doc?id=10118500&ppg=246

* McCarthy GM and McCarty DJ. Effect of topical capsaicin in the therapy of painful osteoarthritis of the hands. J Rheumatol 1992; 19:604– 607.

* McAlindon TE, Jacques P, Zhang Y et al. Do antioxidant micronutrients protect against the development and progression on knee osteoarthritis? Arth Rheum 1996:39(4); 648– 656.

* Pipitone VR. Chondroprotection with chondroitin sulfate. Drugs Exp Clin Res 1991; 17:3.

* Morreale P. Comparison of the antiinflammatory efficacy of chondroitin sulfate and diclofenac sodium in patients with knee osteoarthritis. J Rheumatol 1996; 23:1385.

* Adams ME, Atkinson MH, Lussier AJ et al. The role of viscosupplementation with hylan G– F 20 (Synvisc) in the treatment of osteoarthritis of the knee: A Canadian multicenter trial comparing hylan G– F 20 alone, hylan G– F 20 with nonsteroidal antiin-flammatory drugs (NSAIDs) and NSAIDs alone. Osteoarthritis and Cartilage 1995; 3:213– 225.

* Balazs EA and Denlinger JL. Viscosupplementation: A new concept in the treatment of osteoarthritis. J Rheumatol 1993; supp 39; 20:3– 9.

* Leeb BF, Petera P, Neumann K. [Results of a multicenter study of chondroitin sulfate (Condrosulf) use in arthroses of the finger, knee and hip joints] {German}. Wiener Medizinische Wochenschrift 1996; 146:604– 614.

* Barclay TS, Tsourounis C, McCart GM. Glucosamine. Ann Pharmacother 1998; 32:574– 579.

* Drovanti A. Therapeutic activity of oral glucosamine sulfate in osteoarthritis: A placebo-controlled double-blind investigation. Clin Ther 1980; 3:260.

* Qi GX, Gao SN, Giacovelli G et al. Efficacy and safety of glucosamine sulfate versus ibuprofen in patients with knee osteoarthritis. Arzneimittelforschung 1998; 48:469– 474. Vas AL.

* Doubleblind clinical evaluation of the relative efficacy of ibuprofen and glucosamine sulfate in the management of osteoarthritis of the knee in outpatients. Curr Med Res Opin 1982; 8:145– 149.

* Creamer P. Intra-articular corticosteroid injections in osteoarthritis: do they work and if so, how? Ann Rheum Dis 1997; 56:634– 36.

* Scale D, Wobig M, Wolpert W. Viscosupplementation of osteoarthritic knees with hylan: A treatment schedule study. Current Therapeutic Research 1994; 55:220– 232.

* Yasui T, Akatsuka M, Tobetto K. Effects of hyaluronan on the production of stromelysin and tissue inhibitor of mettaloproteinase– 1 in bovine articular chondrocytes. Biomedical Research. 1992; 13:343– 348.

* Tobetto K, Nakai K, Akatsuka M, et al: Inhibitory effects of hyaluronan on neutrophil mediated cartilage degredation. Connect Tissue Res 1993; 29:181– 190.

* Armstrong S, Read R, Ghosh P. The effects of intraarticular hyaluronan on cartilage and subchondral bone changes in an ovine model of early osteoarthritis. J Rhematol. 21:680– 688, 199.

* Brandt KD. Osteoarthritis. In: Harrison's Principles of Internal Medicine. New York: McGraw-Hill, 1994; 13:1692– 1698.

* Minor MA, Hewitt JE, Webel RR et al. Efficacy of physical conditioning exercise on inpatients with RA and OA. Arthritis Rheum 1989; 32:1396– 1405.

* Fisher NM, Pendergast DR, Gresham GE, Calkins E. Muscle rehabilitation: Its effect on muscular and functional performance of patients with knee OA. Arch Phys Med Rehabil 1991; 72:367– 374.

* Ekdahl C, Andersson SI, Moritz V, Svensson B. dynamic v. static training in patients with RA. Scand J Rheumatol 1990; 19: 17– 26.

* Chamberlain MA, Care G, Harfield B. Physiotherapy in osteoarthritis of the knees. A controlled trial of hospital versus home exercises. Int Rehabil Med 1982, 4:101– 106.

* Wobig M, Dickhut A, Maier R et al. Viscosupplementation with hylan G– F 20: A 26– week controlled trial of efficacy and safety in the osteoarthritic knee. Clin Ther 1998; 20:410– 423.

* Creamer P, Sharif M, George E, et al. Intraarticular hyaluronic acid in osteoarthritis of the knee: An investigation into

mechanisms of action. Osteoarthritis and Cartilage, 2; 133– 140, 1994.

* Listrat V, Ayral X, Patarnello F et al. evaluation of the potential structure modifying activity of hyaluronan (hyalgan) in osteoarthritis of the knee. Osteoarthritis and Cartilage. 1997; 5:153– 160.

* Felson DT, Zhang Y, Anthony JM, Naimark A, Anderson JJ. Weight loss reduces the risk for symptomatic osteoarthritis in women. The Framingham Study. Ann Intern Med 1992, 116(7):535– 539. 57. Alpiner NM, Oh TN, Brander VA. Rehabilitation in joint and connective tissue diseases. SAE Study Guide 1995, 76(55) 532.

* VanBaar ME, Assendelft WJ, Dekker J et al. Effectiveness of exercise therapy in patients with osteoarthritis of the hip or knee: a systematic review of randomized clinical trials. J Rheumatol 1998; 25(12); 2432– 2439.

* Kovar PA, Allegrante JP, MacKenzie CR, et al. Supervised fitness walking in patients with osteoarthritis of the knee. Ann Intern Med 1992; 116:529– 534.

* Perlman SG, Connell KJ, Clark A et al. Dance-based aerobic exercise for rheumatoid arthritis. Arthritis Care Res 1990; 3:29– 35.

* Semble EL, Loeser RF, Wise CM. Therapeutic exercise for rheumatoid arthritis and osteoarthritis. Semin Arthritis Rheum 1990; 20:32– 40.

* Byers PH. Effect of exercise on morning stiffness and mobility in patients with rheumatoid arthritis. Res Nurs Health 1985; 8:275– 281.

* Feinberg J, Marzouk D, Sokolek C, Katz B, Bradley J, Brandt K. Effects of isometric versus range of motion exercises on joint pain and function in patients with knee osteoarthritis (abstract). Arth Rheum 1992, 35 (Suppl 5): R28.

* Keefe FJ and Caldwell DS. Cognitive behavioral control of arthritis pain. Med Clinics N Am 1997; 81:277– 290.

* Keefe FJ, Caldwell DS, Williams DA et al. Pain coping skills training in the management of osteoarthritic knee pain: A comparative study. Behav Ther 1990; 21:49– 62.

* Lorig KR, Mazonson PD, Holman HR. Evidence suggesting that health education for self-management in patients with chronic arthritis sustained health benefits while reducing health care costs. Arthritis Rheum 1993; 36: 439– 446.

* Weinberger M, Tierney WM, Cowpar PA et al. Cost-effectiveness of increased telephone contact for patients with osteoarthritis: A randomized controlled trial. Arthritis Rheum 1993; 36:243– 246.

* Nicholas JJ, Gruen H et al. Splinting in rheumatoid arthritis. I. Factors affecting patient compliance. Arch Phys Med Rehab 63:92– 94, 1982.

* Falconer J, Hayes, KW, Chang, RW. Effect of ultrasound on mobility in osteoarthritis of the knee. A radomized clinical trial. Arth Care Res 5:29– 35, 1992.

* Chang RW, Falconer J, Stulberg SD et al. A randomized controlled trial of arthroscopic surgery versus closed needle lavage for patients with osteoarthritis of the knee. Arth Rheum 1993; 36:289– 296.

* Harris WH and Sledge CB. Total hip and total knee replacement, parts 1 and 2. N Eng J Med 1990; 323:725– 31, 801– 807.

* Chang RW, Pellissier JM, Hazen GB. A cost-effectiveness analysis of total hip arthroplasty for osteoarthritis of the hip. JAMA 1996; 275:858– 865.

* Brander VA, Malhotra S, Jet J et al. Outcome of hip and knee arthroplasty in persons aged 80 years and older. Clin Ortho Rel Res 1997; 345:67– 78.

* Wilder RL. Rheumatoid arthritis: epidemiology, pathology and pathogenesis. In: Schumacher HR, Klippel JH, Koopman WJ (eds.), Primer on the Rheumatic Diseases, 10th edition. Atlanta: Arthritis Foundation, 1993, 86– 89.

* Pincus T, Callahan LF. Reassessment of twelve traditional paradigms concerning the diagnosis, prevalence, morbidity, and mortality of rheumatoid arthritis. Scan J Rheum 1989, Suppl.79:67.

* Pincus T, Callahan LF. Early mortality in rheumatoid arthritis predicted by poor clinical status. Bull Rheum Dis 1992; 41:4.

* Wilske KR, Healy LA. Remodeling the pyramid: A concept whose time has come. J Rheumatol 1989; 16(5):565– 567.

* Elliot MJ, Maini RN, Feldmann M. Repeated therapy with monoclonal antibody to TNFa (cA2) in patients with RA. Lancet 1994; 344:1125– 1127.

* Group GLS. Double-blind controlled Phase III multicenter clinical trial with interferon gamma in rheumatoid arthritis. Rheumatol Int 1992:12:175– 185.

* Hawley DJ, Wolfe F. Anxiety and depression in patients with rheumatoid arthritis: A prospective study of 400 patients. J Rheumatol 1988; 15:932– 941.

* Katz PP, Yelin EH. The development of depressive symptoms among women with RA: The role of function. Arthritis Rheum 1995; 38: 49– 56.

* Hagglund HJ, Haley WE, Reveille JD, Alarcon GS. Predicting individual differences in pain and functional impairment among patients with RA. Arthritis Rheum 1989; 32:851– 858.

* Frank RG, Hagglund KJ. Mood Disorders. In: Wegener ST, Belza BL, Gall EP (eds.), Clinical Care in the Rheumatic Diseases. Atlanta: American College of Rheumatology, 1996:125– 130.

* Gerber LH. Exercise and arthritis. Bull Rheum Dis 1990; 39:1– 9.

* Nordemar R. Physical training in rheumatoid arthritis: a controlled long-term study. II. Functional capacity and general attitudes. Scand J Rheum 1981; 10:25– 30.

* Nordemar R, Ekblom B, Zachrisson L et al. Physical training in rheumatoid arthritis: A controlled long-term study. I. Functional capacity and general attitudes. Scand J Rheum 1981; 10:17– 23.

* Hicks SE. Exercise in patients with inflammatory arthritis and connective tissue disease. Rheum Dis Clinics NA 1990; 16(4):845.

* Clark SR, Burckhardt CS, Bennett RM. Exercise for prevention and treatment of illness. In Exercise for prevention and treatment of illness.

* Basmajian JV and Wolf SL. In: Gerber LH, Hicks JE (eds.), Therapeutic Exercise, 5th edition. Baltimore: Williams and Wilkins, 1990; 340.

* Herbison GJ, Ditunno Jr, Jaweed MM. Muscle atrophy in rheumatoid arthritis. J Rheumatol 1987; S15(14):78– 81.

* Lefebvre JC, KeefeFJ, Affleck G et al. The relationship of arthritis self-efficacy to daily pain, daily mood, and daily pain coping in rheumatoid arthritis patients. Pain 1999; 80:425– 435.

* Parker JC, Smarr KL, Buckelew SP et al. Effects of stress management on clinical outcomes in rheumatoid arthritis. Arthritis Rheum 1995; 38:1807– 1818.

* Williams J, Harvey J, Tannenbaum H. Use of superficial heat versus ice for thc rheumatoid arthritic shoulder: A pilot study. Physiotherapy Canada 38:8– 13, 1986.

* Green J, McKenna F, Redfern EJ, Chamberlain MA: Home exercises are as effective as outpatient hydrotherapy for osteoarthritis of the hip. Br J Rheumatol 32:812– 815, 1993.

* Mainardi CL, Walter JM, Spiegel PK, et al. Rheumatoid arthritis: Failure of daily heat therapy to affect its progression. Arch Phys Med Rehabil 1979:60(9); 390– 393.

* Hashish I, Harvey W, Harris M. Antiinflammatory effects of ultrasound therapy: evidence for major placebo effect. Br J Rheumatol 25:77– 81, 1986.

* Oosterveld FGJ, Rasker JJ< Jacobs JWG, Overmars HJA. The effect of local heat and cold therapy on the intraarticular and skin surface temperature of the knee. Arthritis Rheum 1992; 35:146– 151.

* Kumar VN, Redford JB. Transcutaneous nerve stimulation in rheumatoid arthritis. Arch Phys Med Rehabil 63:75– 78, 1987.

* Hayes KW. Physical Modalities. In: Wegener ST, Belza BL, Gall EP (eds.), Clinical Care in the Rheumatic Diseases. Atlanta: American College of Rheumatology, 1996: 79– 82.

* Partridge REH, Duthie JJR. Controlled trial of the effect of complete immobilization of the joints in rheumatoid arthritis. Ann Rheum Dis 22:91– 99, 1963.

* Gault SJ, Spyker JM: Beneficial effects of immobilization of joints in rheumatoid arthritis and related arthritidities: A splint study using sequencial analysis. Arthritis Rheum 12:34– 44, 1969.

* Boden SD. Rheumatoid arthritis of the cervical spine. Surgical decision making based on predictors of paralysis and recovery. Spine 1994; 19(20):2275– 2280.

* Goldberg, VM, Figgie HE, Inglis AE, Figgie MP. Current concepts review: Total elbow arthroplasty. J Bone Joint Surg 1988; 70– A:778– 783. Jolly SL, Ferlic DC, Clayton ML, Dennis DA, Stringer EA. Swanson silicone arthroplasty of wrist in rheumatoid arthritis: A long-term follow-up. J Hand Surg 1992:17:142– 149.

Note: Source for images: ***httpwww.gettyimages.com***

Made in the USA
Monee, IL
04 November 2026

67380799R00085